THE CARE
TRAINING OF THE
MENTALLY SUBNORMAL

BY

CHARLES H. HALLAS

S.R.N., R.M.N., R.N.M.S., R.N.T.

Head of Nursing Services, Lancaster Moor Hospital; Formerly Principal Nursing Officer, Lynebank Hospital, Dunfermline; Examiner for the General Nursing Council for Scotland; Chief Male Nurse, Brentry Hospital, Westbury-on-Trym, Bristol; Examiner for the General Nursing Council

WITH A FOREWORD BY

RONALD C. MACGILLIVRAY

M.B., Ch.B. (Edin.), F.R.C.P. (Glas.), D.P.M. (Lond.)

Lecturer on Mental Deficiency in the University of Glasgow; Physician Superintendent, Lennox Castle

FOURTH EDITION

BRISTOL: JOHN WRIGHT & SONS LTD.

1970

Distribution by Sole Agents
United States of America: The Williams & Wilkins Company, Baltimore
Canada: The Macmillan Company of Canada, Ltd., Toronto

First Edition, March, 1958 (" The Nursing of Mental Defectives ")
Second Edition, November, 1962 (" Nursing the Mentally Subnormal ")
Third Edition, February, 1967 ("The Care and Training of the Mentally Subnormal")
Fourth Edition, November, 1970

ISBN 0 7236 0266 2

PRINTED IN GREAT BRITAIN BY JOHN WRIGHT & SONS LTD.
AT THE STONEBRIDGE PRESS, BRISTOL BS4 5NU

PREFACE TO THE FOURTH EDITION

PROFESSIONALLY we have maintained that the mentally subnormal patient should be better served through improved standards in the selection of candidates for training in our schools of nursing.

The education of the student nurse should be improved to keep in step with the advance in medical knowledge. Nurse education must be reorganized to meet the advancing ideas for the prevention of mental subnormality and the promotion of rehabilitative methods and community care.

To meet the increasing demands for more nurses, a larger number of untrained personnel has been introduced into the nursing establishments of hospitals and allocated to wards and departments without any introduction to nursing care, training, and nursing ethics. We cannot and should not dismiss these facts from our considerations.

As a profession we should resist the continued pressures to lower the standard of nursing, but insist that everyone has a minimum period of instruction before joining a nursing team and that regular annual refresher courses are made available for all nurses. This is the only way we can be sure that the patient's needs will be adequately catered for.

I would like to think that this fourth edition will be an aid towards a better standard of care and training for the mentally subnormal patient.

' But for the Grace of God, there go I. '

CHARLES H. HALLAS

October, 1970

CONTENTS

FOREWORD

By Ronald C. MacGillivray

M.B., Ch.B. (Edin.), F.R.C.P. (Glas.), D.P.M. (Lond.)

Lecturer on Mental Deficiency in the University of Glasgow;
Physician Superintendent, Lennox Castle

It is a pleasant task for me to write a few words as a foreword to this excellent book. For years the public, teachers, nurses, and the medical profession have regarded mental subnormality as an uninteresting, unrewarding, not quite respectable backwater which dealt with unattractive patients for whom little could be done. Some hospital staffs lived in deplorable isolation while too many general nurses looked down on their mental nurse colleagues whose job was not always regarded as 'proper nursing'. Nor indeed did ignorant administrators appreciate fully the special needs of the hospitals for the mentally subnormal. An inevitable result has been the welter of unfortunate controversy which surrounds the mental deficiency services today.

The public generally have been disinterested in this thankless work, apart from a certain enthusiasm for witch-hunts when some overtaxed nurse falls from grace. The rest of the time they have brushed the mentally retarded under the carpet like human dust and indeed many of the measures now proposed only represent a salve to the public conscience and provide little real benefit to the mentally subnormal.

In subnormality nursing, as in medicine generally, there is an especially urgent need for a sound scientific approach. This is necessary as a basis both for the education of the handicapped and also for the care of patients. Without such objective classification the scientific basis of mental deficiency is just as impossible as the rational treatment of disease would be without knowledge of the nature of the illness and the clinical state of the patient.

As long ago as 1866, the publishing firm of Longmans, Green & Co., of London, issued *A Manual for the Classification,*

Training and Education of the Feeble-minded, Imbecile and Idiotic. In the introduction the authors, Duncan and Millard, deplore the paucity of background material for their monograph. A century has passed and still the essential nursing data, though less scarce, are scattered, some buried in journals or pamphlets, some carried along by tradition as legends, and some concerned with specific fragmentary details.

This book by Charles Hallas is distinguished from many other writings in the field by its breadth of scope and by the careful and systematic nature of the contents. The many additions which have been made to the general store of knowledge concerning mental retardation in the past few years have necessitated a complete revision of the last edition. Much new material has been included, parts have been virtually rewritten, and the book emphasizes realism and positive action in the nursing of the subnormal in contrast to the outlook of hopeless resignation which still too often prevails.

It will continue to be of great assistance to mental deficiency nurses in England and Scotland, and, whilst primarily written for these, is valuable to social workers, to health visitors, to undergraduate and postgraduate students of medicine, and to all whose work brings them in contact with the subnormality field from time to time.

If one further takes into account the human and optimistic approach with which the author tackles the problem, the importance of this book becomes clear. No one can doubt that a reader who acquaints himself with it will come to value the clarity of thought and approve of the motives which inspired the author in so important a work.

THE CARE AND TRAINING OF
THE MENTALLY SUBNORMAL

CHAPTER I

INTRODUCTORY

EVER since men began to live in communities they have faced the problem of dealing with those who do not ' fit in '. Some could be tolerated, but others, in early days, were locked away or put to death.

As society became more complex, the number of misfits became even greater, and their existence more of a problem. The hospital for the mentally subnormal is the result of early attempts to care for those who, because of mental defect, are unable to take a normal place in society.

It was not until the middle of the nineteenth century that any attempt was made to face the problem. Some Christian communities had previously provided shelter for a small number, but harsh treatment only was the lot of the majority.

A Frenchman, Dr. Itard, was among the first to try to train and educate the mentally subnormal. His early efforts (1800) were carried out on a boy he found wandering, whom he called the " Savage of Aveyron ". As a result, and through the continued enthusiasm of Dr. Edouard Séquin, one of Dr. Itard's students, twenty-four schools and institutions were opened.

For the next few years various attempts were made to cure the mentally subnormal, but no general system of permanent care and control was evolved. After a period in special schools, the patient was discharged into society again, in the same condition as when he first left it. Finally, the truth dawned that there was no cure for these patients, but more important still was the realization of the numbers of these maladjusted beings in the community.

After abortive curative experiments the public became alarmed over the number of mentally subnormal people in their midst. The mentally subnormal person was blamed for many social evils, and because of this, permanent segregation in institutions was demanded.

THE AIMS OF THE HOSPITAL

In caring for and encouraging the mentally subnormal patient, the nurse will require a definite philosophy of optimism and faith to guide her in her work. It is important that she be dominated by a certainty that even the severest retardation will yield to reconditioning. The road to rehabilitation will be hard and difficult for her, and one which will demand self-discipline and determination for the upward climb.

First, the nurse and the patient must be willing to tackle the task of overcoming the difficulties together with willingness and assurance. Later, the nurse, the social worker, and the parents, with the patient may achieve the thrilling objective of rehabilitation.

A large number of patients living in the hospital are there for reasons of unpleasant conduct, which may have arisen from their family circumstances or their innate defects. In other words, they are in hospital because they cannot live in society and society will not tolerate them.

In the rehabilitation of a person of this kind there are six groups of people taking part: (1) Medical staff; (2) Nursing staff; (3) Teaching staff; (4) Occupational Therapy staff; (5) Psychologists ; (6) Social workers.

The primary need of all human beings is to be loved, valued, and appreciated as an individual. In mentally subnormal persons the parents first take on the responsibility, followed later by the nursing staff, who take over the parental function immediately the patient is admitted to their care. In emotionally disturbed patients who may have suffered emotional deprivation, and whose behaviour is antagonistic, this need of love is very great. The nurse must therefore meet this need, and also be prepared to appreciate and respond continually to the changing requirements of the individual patient.   Sooner or later because of this care the patient will respond by having confidence in the nurse.

The human values and emotional needs of the patients should be assessed individually, and not calculated on the fact that patients have the same calendar age (chronological age) and mental age.   Work, gifts, and pleasures must be matched to the capacity and interest of the patient.

New and more hopeful attitudes towards the mentally subnormal patient are making it increasingly more important for the hospitals to re-examine their own functions and aims. In the past, segregation and efficient care were all that was considered necessary and minimum standards were all that was usually given.   Now the hospital for the mentally subnormal person must serve the following purposes:—

1. A training school to provide education for all mentally subnormal patients who are unable to benefit from training outside suited to their needs.

2. A place of shelter for those in need of care and protection.

3. A hospital for those who require special nursing care because of physical deformities or severe degrees of subnormality.

4. A place of control for those who are a danger to themselves and others and who may be in need of psychotherapy treatment.

5. A place of preparation for future community care, where the patient is taught to make a satisfactory social adjustment as far as his degree of subnormality will allow.

The aims, therefore, can be summarized as follows: to help the patient to live a happy life within the hospital; direction on how to form good habits and attitudes; development of individual abilities, interests, and aptitudes, and of favourable personal characteristics; interest and proficiency at work; and encouragement in thinking for himself and solving some of his own problems without the aid of the nurse.

The patient should be encouraged to form a code of ethical behaviour and be willing to help his neighbour who is less able to care for himself.   If a sense of being needed and of belonging can be imbued into the patient much will have been achieved. Self-control, respect for other people's property, and ability to accept responsibility should be amongst the aims of the hospital.

It is essential that the nurse should realize the great importance of the development of her powers of observation in her work. Her ability to notice the smallest of changes in her patient, who is unable to convey his feelings to her, will be of great value to his welfare, the doctor's information, and her own interest.

The Pioneer Spirit.—Every hospital has room for the nurse possessing this quality. Though it is not an essential qualification for caring for the mentally subnormal, it can be invaluable both to the patient and the hospital. New ideas will not readily be accepted. Intensive opposition, even from the patients, will result from any change of routine if every member involved has not had the opportunity for studying and discussing the proposed change. The resistance will not be malicious, but there is security in doing something we understand: the end result is known and the patient is no worse off; but with a changed and new routine there is an immediate sense of discomfort and insecurity resulting from the unknown. If the nurse and patient can be persuaded to accept the change before it is brought into force, everyone will approach it with a will to make it a success.

When there are good staff relationships the senior nurse will not feel resentment if a nurse junior to herself has put forward a new idea. The ward sister or charge nurse will welcome a situation in which all members of the nursing staff feel free to suggest changes from which possible benefits may occur.

CHAPTER II

LEGAL ASPECTS OF MENTAL SUBNORMALITY

IN 1954 a Royal Commission was set up to inquire into conditions within mental hospitals and hospitals for mental defectives, and on the law relating to this branch of medicine. As a result of this a new Act was placed before Parliament in 1959, which became law in 1960, the year which had been declared as Mental Health Year.

Three important principles receive emphasis in the new Act :—

1. That as much treatment as possible in and out of hospital shall be given as a voluntary measure, and that it will be as easy for the mentally disordered patient to obtain treatment in a suitable hospital as it is for the physically ill person.

2. That, where possible, treatment and training will be available in the community for all those patients who are not needing hospital care but who are able to live in their own homes or in a special home or hostel.

3. Only those who are ill enough to require care and treatment for their own sakes or for the sake of their families and the community and who are unwilling to go to hospital are now subject to any kind of compulsion. In such cases the recommendation of two doctors is all that is necessary. However, to safeguard such patients from any risk of being kept in hospital unnecessarily each Regional Hospital Board has been empowered to provide a special tribunal to which patients or their relatives can appeal for a review of their case at certain phases of the detention period.

Prior to the inception of the new Act there were many mental defectives who had spent many years in hospital because they had nowhere else to go and needed a certain amount of help and care. They did not require hospital treatment and would have been much happier and less likely to deteriorate mentally had they been allowed to live a more normal life and have a measure of independence in their own homes or in small hostels. A number of younger ones could have gone out to work and become self-supporting to some extent.

One of the redeeming features of the new Act is that the relatively few laws that apply to mentally subnormal people apply only to the very small minority who are subject to detention orders.

Local authorities have been given greater powers to provide preventive and after-care services as well as community care for those patients who do not need to be treated or detained in hospital. This will apply to adults and children.

The Mental Deficiency Act, 1913.—This Act made permanent care both possible and legal. It was the first real effort to do something for the mentally subnormal, and was so complete that only slight amendments have had to be made since. However, the modern approach to mental disorder rendered the 1913 Act unacceptable.

The Mental Health Act, 1959 is a completely new approach to the administrative problem of treatment, if necessary under compulsion, of mental patients and mental defectives, now known as mentally disordered persons.

Classification of Mental Disorder.—In the Mental Health Act, mental disorder means:—

  1. Mental illness.
  2. Arrested or incomplete development of the mind.
  3. Psychopathic disorder.
  4. Any other disorder or disability of the mind.

The classifications and definitions of mental subnormality are:—

  1. *Severe Subnormality.*—A state of arrested or incomplete development of the mind which includes subnormality of the intelligence and is of such a nature or degree that the patient is incapable of living an independent life or of guarding himself against serious exploitation, or will be so incapable when of an age to do so.

  2. *Subnormality.*—A state of arrested or incomplete development of mind, not amounting to severe subnormality, which

includes subnormality of intelligence, and is of a nature or degree which requires, or is susceptible to, medical treatment or other special care or training of the patient.

3. *Psychopathic Disorder.*—A persistent disorder or disability of mind, whether or not including subnormality of intelligence, which results in abnormally aggressive or seriously irresponsible conduct on the part of the patient and requires, or is susceptible to, medical treatment.

Section 1.—The Mental Health Act, 1959 repealed the Lunacy and Mental Treatment Acts, 1890–1930 and the Mental Deficiency Acts, 1913–1938, and made fresh provisions for the care and treatment of mentally disordered persons and the management of their property and affairs.

Section 2.—The Board of Control was also dissolved.

Section 3.—*Mental Health Review Tribunals.* To each Regional Hospital Board Area there is one Mental Health Review Tribunal. Each Tribunal must consist of:—

1. A number of legal members approved by the Lord Chancellor.

2. A number of medical members appointed by the Lord Chancellor after consultation with the Minister.

3. A number of administrators who have experience of Social Services. The Chairman of the Tribunal must be a legal member.

Section 122.—*Powers and proceeding of Mental Health Review Tribunals.* All applications to the Mental Health Review Tribunals have to be made in writing to the appropriate Tribunal for the area in which the patient is residing either in hospital, or nursing home, or under guardianship.

Section 123.—Where an application has been made to a Mental Health Review Tribunal in respect of a patient liable to be detained, the Tribunal may direct that the patient be discharged if they are satisfied that the patient is not suffering from mental illness, psychopathic disorder, subnormality, or severe subnormality, or that it is not necessary in the interests of his health or safety or for the protection of others for him to be detained, and that he is not likely to act in a manner dangerous to other persons or himself. The Tribunal may also direct that a patient under guardianship be discharged.

Section 28.—The application for admission. An application for admission has to be based on the written recommendations on the prescribed form signed by two Medical Practitioners who have personally examined the patient.

One of the Medical Practitioners must be approved for the purpose as having special experience in the diagnosis or treatment of mental disorder by the Local Health Authority. If practicable, the other recommendation should be given by a Medical Practitioner who has acquaintance with the patient.

Section 30.—Application for admission in respect of a patient already in hospital. If in the case of a patient who is an in-patient in a hospital and not liable to be detained and it appears to the responsible medical officer that an application for admission to hospital is necessary, he should furnish to the Managers a report in writing to that effect. In such a case, the patient may be detained in the hospital for a period of 3 days. The object of this provision is to allow time for an application for admission to be made.

Section 33.—Guardianship. A guardianship application may be made in respect of a patient on the grounds that:—

1. He is suffering from mental disorder, this being:—

a. In the case of a patient of any age, mental illness or severe subnormality.

b. In the case of a patient under the age of 21 years, psychopathic disorder or subnormality, and that his disorder is of a nature or degree which warrants the reception of the patient into guardianship, and

2. It is necessary in the interests of the patient or for the protection of other persons that the patient should be so received.

The application must be supported by two medical recommendations. The person named as guardian may be either a Local Health Authority, or any other person including the applicant.

*Section 34.—*The application for guardianship has to be forwarded to the Local Health Authority within 14 days, beginning with the day the patient was last examined by a Medical Practitioner before giving medical recommendation.

If the application is accepted by the Local Health Authority, the application immediately confers on the named guardian the same powers over the patient as would be the case if he were the father of the patient and the patient were under the age of 14 years. The patient may apply to a Mental Health Review Tribunal within a period of 6 months beginning with the day on which the application is accepted, or with the day on which he attains the age of 16 years whichever is the later.

Section 5.—Informal admission. A mentally subnormal person may be admitted informally to any hospital or nursing home for treatment for mental disorder. A patient under the age of 16 years may be detained in hospital at his parents' or guardians' request, no matter what his wishes are. On reaching the age of 16 years and expressing his wish to leave the hospital, he may leave the hospital irrespective of the wishes of his parents or guardians.

Compulsory Admission to Hospital.—

Section 25.—Admission for observation. A patient may be detained for observation with or without treatment for a period not exceeding 28 days, providing it can be shown that he is suffering from a mental disorder which warrants his detention in the interests of his own health and safety or for the protection of others.

Section 26.—Admission for treatment. Application for admission for treatment may be made in respect of a patient on the grounds that:—

He is suffering from mental disorder,

a. In the case of a patient of any age, mental illness or severe subnormality,

b. In the case of a patient under the age of 21 years, psychopathic disorder or subnormality,

of such a degree that it warrants his detention in hospital for medical treatment in the interests of the patient's health or safety, or for the protection of other persons.

The detention may be for a period not exceeding 1 year in the first instance.

Section 29.—Admission for observation in case of emergency. In the case of emergency, the Mental Welfare Officer or any relative of the patient may make application for admission and detention in hospital for observation under Section 25. If going through the full procedure would involve unreasonable delay the application may be founded on one medical certificate but such application will cease to have effect after the expiration of 72 hours, unless a second medical recommendation is received by the Managers.

Section 60.—Admission of patients concerned in criminal proceedings and transfer of patients under sentence. Where a person is convicted before a Court of Assize, or Quarter Sessions (in the case of a person convicted of an offence other than an offence for which the sentence is fixed by law), or a Magistrates' Court (in the case of a person convicted of an offence punishable on summary conviction with imprisonment), and the Court, being satisfied with the written or oral evidence of two Medical Practitioners that the person is suffering from mental illness, psychopathic disorder, subnormality, or severe subnormality, and the mental disorder is of a nature or degree which warrants his detention in hospital, or reception into guardianship, may order this form of care.

The Court must be satisfied that the hospital specified will be able to admit the patient within a period of 28 days or that the Local Health Authority or other person specified is willing to receive the patient into guardianship.

A Magistrates' Court may make an Order under this Section of the Act without convicting a person suffering from mental illness or severe subnormality, provided the Court is satisfied he committed the act.

Section 61.—If a child or young person is brought before a Juvenile Court and the Court is satisfied that the child or young person is in need of care and protection, or that his parent or guardian is unable to control him, it may make a hospital or guardianship Order. Before making the Order the Court must be satisfied that the parent or guardian understands the results which will follow from the Order, and that they consent to its being made.

Leave of Absence from Hospital.—

Section 39.—The Responsible Medical Officer may grant for any period leave of absence from hospital to a patient detained in hospital, subject to such conditions as the Officer considers necessary. A patient to whom leave of absence is granted shall not be recalled to hospital after he has ceased to be liable to be detained in hospital or after the expiration of 6 months, unless he has returned to the hospital.

Absence Without Leave.—

Section 40.—If a patient, who is liable to be detained in hospital, absents himself from the hospital without permission or fails to return to the hospital on expiration of any leave, he may be taken into custody and returned to hospital by any Mental Welfare Officer; by any Officer on the staff of the hospital; by any Constable or by any person authorized in writing by the Managers of the hospital. Patients subject to guardianship are dealt with in the same way.

Psychopathic and subnormal patients over the age of 21 years, on the first day of absence without leave, may be dealt with in this way at any time within a period of 6 months, beginning with that day. In other cases this period is limited to 28 days. After these periods have expired, the patient ceases to be liable to be detained or subject to guardianship.

Transfer of Patients.—

Section 41.—A patient who is liable to be detained in hospital, or subject to guardianship, may be transferred to another hospital or into guardianship of another Local Health Authority. The transfer of the patient from hospital to guardianship, or vice versa, is permissible.

A patient, who, having attained the age of 16 years, is transferred from guardianship to a hospital, may apply to the Mental Health Review Tribunal within the period of 6 months.

Duration of Authority for Detention or Guardianship and Discharge of Patients.—

Section 43.—The period of detention in hospital or under guardianship is limited to a period not exceeding 1 year. Authority for detention or guardianship may be renewed for a further period of 1 year and from the expiration of this further period any further renewals are for periods of 2 years. A report recommending continued detention should be furnished to the Managers by the Responsible Medical Officer, or to the Local Health Authority by the nominated medical attendant of a patient under guardianship, stating that continued detention is necessary in the interests of the patient's health or safety, or for the protection of others, and the authority for continued detention is thereby renewed.

The Managers or Local Health Authority must notify patients over the age of 16 years of each renewal of authority, and the patient may apply to a Mental Health Review Tribunal within the period for which the authority is renewed.

Section 44.—Upon attaining the age of 25 years, the authority for the detention or guardianship of a psychopathic or subnormal patient will cease to have effect unless in the case of a patient detained in hospital the Responsible Medical Officer, within the period of 2 months ending on the patient's 25th birthday, furnishes to the Managers a report that it appears to him that the patient would be likely to act in a manner dangerous to other persons or to himself if released from hospital. When such a report is furnished, the Managers are required to inform the patient and nearest relative who have the right within a period of 28 days, beginning with the patient's 25th birthday, to apply to the Mental Health Review Tribunal.

Discharge of Patients.—

Section 47.—Orders for discharge may be made by:—

1. The Responsible Medical Officer, or the Managers of the hospital in the case of a patient detained for observation.

2. The Responsible Medical Officer, the Managers of the hospital, or the nearest relative in the case of a patient detained for treatment.

3. The Responsible Medical Officer, the responsible Local Health Authority, or the nearest relative in the case of a patient subject to guardianship.

Additional Authorities for Discharge.—

1. The registration authority in the case of a patient liable to be detained in a Mental Nursing Home for observation or treatment.

2. The Regional Hospital Board, if the patient is maintained under a contract with the Board.

Restriction on Discharge by the Nearest Relative.—

Section 48.—The nearest relative must give at least 72 hours' notice in writing to the Managers of his wish to discharge the patient. If the Responsible Medical Officer reports to the Managers within the period of notice that in his opinion the patient would be likely to be dangerous to others or himself if discharged, they may continue his detention against his nearest relative's wish. In this case the nearest relative may not order discharge during the next 6 months. The Managers must inform the relative of the report, and their right to apply to a Mental Health Review Tribunal within a period of 28 days.

Where a report has been furnished by the Responsible Medical Officer that a psychopathic or subnormal patient having attained the age of 25 years would be likely to act in a manner dangerous to others or himself if released, then an Order for discharge may not be made by the nearest relative for a period of 6 months, beginning with the date of that report.

Section 52.—In certain circumstances the functions of the nearest relative may be transferred to any specified person who, in the opinion of the County Court, is a proper person to act as the patient's nearest relative, and is willing to do so, and such an application may be made by:—

1. Any relative of the patient.

2. Any other person with whom the patient is residing, or was last residing with before admission to hospital.

3. A Mental Welfare Officer.

The nearest relative of this patient has the right to apply to a Mental Health Review Tribunal within the period of 12 months beginning with the date of the Order and in any subsequent period of 12 months.

The grounds upon which an Order may be made under this Section are:—

1. That the patient has no nearest relative.

2. That the nearest relative of the patient is incapable of acting as such by reason of mental disorder or other illness.

3. That the nearest relative of the patient unreasonably objects to the making of an application for admission for treatment or a guardianship application in respect of the patient.

4. That the nearest relative of the patient has exercised, without due regard to the welfare of the patient or the interests

of the public, his power to discharge the patient from hospital or guardianship.

Orders Restricting Discharge.—

Section 65.—Where a hospital Order is made in respect of an offender by a Court of Assize or Quarter Sessions, and it appears to the Court having regard to the nature of the offence that there is risk of his committing further offences if set at large, the Court may order special restrictions either with or without a time limit or during such period as may be specified in the Order called "Order Restricting Discharge". Such an Order may not be made unless at least one of the Medical Practitioners gives oral evidence before the Court. Such patients cannot appeal to a Mental Health Review Tribunal, and they can only be discharged or transferred to another hospital with the consent of the Secretary of State.

Section 63.—Relatives of a patient, who is admitted to a hospital or placed under guardianship by virtue of an Order of Court, may not exercise their power to order the patient's discharge. The Order also removes the age limits to the detention of psychopathic and subnormal patients in hospital or under guardianship. A patient admitted under a hospital or guardianship Order may apply to a Mental Health Review Tribunal within a period of 6 months, beginning with the date of the Order or with the day on which he attains the age of 16 years, whichever is the later. His relatives may make a similar application within the period of 12 months, beginning with the date of the Order and in any subsequent period of 12 months.

Section 66.—The Secretary of State, on being satisfied that an Order restricting the discharge of a patient is no longer necessary for the protection of the public, may terminate the Restriction Order. He may also discharge the patient either absolutely or subject to conditions, and in the latter case, to recall him to hospital at any time while the Order restricting discharge is still in force.

The Secretary of State is required to refer to a Mental Health Review Tribunal for their advice within 2 months of receiving a written request to do so from the patient whose Restriction Order has been in force for a year or more. The patient may apply to the Tribunal once during each period during which he could have applied to them had the order restricting his discharge not been in force. However, a patient recalled to hospital after being conditionally discharged may, in addition, make a request to the Secretary of State 6 months after the date of his recall to hospital.

Section 67.—Any person over the age of 14 years convicted by a Magistrates' Court of an offence punishable by imprisonment, and it appears to the Magistrates that a Restriction Order should be made, they may commit him in custody to Quarter Sessions to be dealt with. The Court of Quarter Sessions may make a hospital Order with or without an Order restricting discharge or deal with him in such a way that the Magistrates' Court might have done.

Section 68.—The Magistrates' Court may order the patient's admission to hospital instead of committing him in custody until his case is dealt with by Quarter Sessions. The Order restricts the patient's discharge.

Section 69.—Where an Order restricting discharge is made, the patient may appeal to the Court of Criminal Appeal against the Order.

Section 70.—A patient subjected to a hospital or guardianship Order made by a Magistrates' Court may appeal against the Order to the Quarter Sessions. A child or young person brought before a Juvenile Court as in need of care and protection or as beyond control of his parent or guardian may also appeal to the Quarter Sessions against any Order the Court may make. His parent or guardian may also appeal.

Transfer to Hospital or Guardianship of Prisoners, etc.—

Section 72.—The Secretary of State, being satisfied by reports of at least two Medical Practitioners, one of whom is approved for the purpose by the Local Health Authority, that a person serving a sentence of imprisonment is suffering from mental illness, psychopathic disorder, subnormality, or severe subnormality, and that the mental disorder warrants the patient's detention in hospital for medical treatment, may authorize his transfer to hospital.

A direction under this Section of the Act shall cease to have effect at the expiration of the period of 14 days beginning with the date on which it is given unless within that period the person with respect to whom it was given has been received into the specified hospital.

Section 75.—The transfer of a patient back to prison may be authorized by the Secretary of State on notification by the Responsible Medical Officer that he no longer needs treatment for mental disorder, providing his prison sentence has not expired.

Section 79.—The Secretary of State may order the reception into guardianship of a child or young person detained in an approved school, if he is satisfied that the child is suffering from mental illness, psychopathic disorder, subnormality, or severe subnormality, and that it is in the public interest.

LOCAL AUTHORITY SERVICES

Section 10.—When a mentally disordered child or young person whose rights and powers of his parent are vested in the Local Authority or Local Health Authority is admitted to hospital or nursing home, the Children's Department of the Local Authority has to arrange for visits to be made to him on their behalf and to take any other steps as would be expected to be taken by his parent, whilst he is in hospital.

Section 11.—*Care and training of children in lieu of education.* A duty is imposed upon the Local Education Authority to ascertain what children in their area are suffering from a disability of mind of such a nature or extent as to make them unsuitable for education at school and to serve notice in writing to the parents of any child who has attained the age of 2 years to submit the child for examination by a Medical Officer of the Authority.

The parent may appeal to the Minister of Education against the decision of the Authority within a period of 21 days.

Section 12.—The Local Health Authority is empowered to compel the regular attendance at a training centre, either daily or on a residential basis, of any child of compulsory school age ascertained by the Local Education Authority as being unsuitable for education at school.

The parents may appeal against this decision.

SPECIAL HOSPITALS

Section 97.—The Minister provides such Institutions as appears to him necessary for patients requiring treatment under special security conditions, on account of their dangerous, violent, or criminal propensities.

Section 98.—The special hospitals are under the control and management of the Minister.

Section 99.—Any patient who for the time being is liable to be detained in a special hospital may, at the direction of the Minister, be removed into any other special hospital or any other type of hospital.

LEGAL POSITION OF THE MENTALLY SUBNORMAL

Section 126.—*Ill-treatment.* Ill-treatment may include corporal punishment, causing physical or mental pain, and wilful neglect. No nurse or any other person employed in a hospital or mental nursing home or any of the Managers responsible for the care and treatment of mentally disordered patients shall ill-treat them. It is also an offence for any individual to ill-treat or wilfully neglect a mentally disordered person while he is subject to his guardianship under the Act, or in his custody or care. The penalty for this may be a term of imprisonment, not exceeding 6 months, on summary conviction, or a fine not exceeding £100, or both. Or on conviction on indictment, a term of imprisonment not exceeding 2 years, or a fine, or both.

Section 127.—*Carnal knowledge.* It is illegal for a man to have sexual relationship with any female suffering from severe subnormality, providing he knows or has reason to suspect her to be severely subnormal.

Section 128.—It is an offence for an Officer on the staff of a hospital or mental nursing home or any of the Managers to have sexual intercourse on hospital premises with a woman receiving treatment, either as an in-patient or as an out-patient.

It is also an offence for a man to have unlawful sexual intercourse with a patient subject to his guardianship. In each case it must be shown that the man knew or had reason to suspect that the woman was a mentally disordered person.

3

The penalty for this offence on conviction or indictment is a term of imprisonment, not exceeding 2 years.

Assisting Patients to Absent Themselves Without Leave.—

Section 129.—It is an offence to induce or knowingly assist a patient detained in hospital or subject to guardianship to absent himself without leave or to escape from legal custody or knowingly to harbour a patient absent without leave or prevent him from being taken into custody.

The penalties for the offences are on summary conviction a term of imprisonment not exceeding 6 months, or a fine not exceeding £100, or both, or on conviction on indictment, a term of imprisonment not exceeding 2 years, or a fine, or both.

Warrant to Search For and Remove Patients.—

Section 135.—A Justice of the Peace may issue a Warrant authorizing a Constable to enter, if need be by force, any premises within his jurisdiction, specified in the Warrant, and if thought fit, to remove him to a place of safety with a view to making an application for treatment or care any person if it appears to the Magistrate on information on Oath from a Mental Welfare Officer that there is reasonable cause to suspect that the patient is suffering from mental disorder and to have been ill-treated, neglected, or not kept under proper control or in need of care. The Constable must be accompanied by a Mental Welfare Officer and by a Medical Practitioner.

On sworn evidence of any Constable, a Justice of the Peace may issue a Warrant authorizing any Constable named in the Warrant to enter the premises, if need be by force, to retake and remove the patient to a place of safety. The Constable may be accompanied by a Medical Practitioner and/or the person authorized to take or re-take the patient.

A place of safety as defined in this Section of the Act is:—

1. Accommodation provided by the Local Authority under Part III of the National Health Act, 1940, or
2. Under Part III of the National Assistance Act, 1948.
3. A hospital as defined by the Mental Health Act, 1959.
4. A Police Station.

5. A Mental Nursing Home or residential home for mentally disordered persons.

6. Any other suitable place, the occupier of which is willing to receive the patient temporarily.

If a Constable finds in a public place a person who appears to him to be suffering from mental disorder and to be in immediate need of care or control, the Constable may, if he thinks it necessary for the interest of the patient or for the protection of others, remove him to a place of safety.

A person removed to a place of safety may be detained for a period not exceeding 72 hours, for the purpose of enabling him to be examined by a Medical Practitioner and to be interviewed by a Mental Welfare Officer.

Marriage and Divorce.—There is no law to prevent marriages between mentally subnormal people. Generally speaking these marriages are legal and binding unless the mentally subnormal person who has married can be proved to be incapable of comprehending the nature of the marriage contract, and of fulfilling the physical conditions of marriage. This is a complex subject, however, and each case would need to be considered in the light of its individual circumstances.

Criminal Responsibility.—To be a mentally subnormal person does not free the person from the responsibilities of complying with the laws of the land. If a mentally subnormal person commits a crime, he is still liable to conviction and punishment by law. His mental condition will be investigated by the Court, which may deal with him as a mentally subnormal person, or as a responsible person.

Contracts.—Unless it can be shown that the mentally subnormal person was incapable of comprehending the terms of the contract and that the other person knew that the mental state was such that the mentally subnormal person did not understand the terms of the contract, then the contract entered into is binding.

Testamentary Capacity.—A Will is only valid if the Testator is able, at the time he makes his Will, to recall and keep clearly in his mind: (1) The nature and the extent of his property; (2) The persons who have claims on his bounty; (3) The relative strength of these claims.

Representation of the People Act, 1949, Section 4, Paragraph 3.—A certified mentally subnormal person undergoing hospital care as a detained patient has a legal right to vote, providing his name appears on the Register of Voters for the constituency which includes his place of residence immediately prior to his admission to hospital.

CHAPTER III

CLASSIFICATION OF THE CLINICAL VARIETIES OF MENTAL SUBNORMALITY

THE clinical varieties of mental subnormality may be considered as follows :—

1. **Mental Subnormality following Infections.**—
   a. Gastro-enteritis in the Newborn.
   b. Meningitis.
   c. Congenital Syphilis.
   d. Encephalitis.
   e. Congenital Rubella Syndrome.
   f. Cytomegalic Inclusion Disease.
   g. Toxoplasmosis.

2. **Mental Subnormality following Injury or Physical Agents.**—
   a. Pre-eclampsia and Eclampsia.
   b. Excessive Intra-uterine Irradiation.
   c. Birth Injury.
   d. Rhesus Incompatibility.
   e. Drugs and the Newborn.
   f. Lead Poisoning.

3. **Mental Subnormality associated with Disorders of Metabolism.**—
   a. Disorders of Lipid Metabolism.—
      i. Amaurotic Family Idiocy (cerebromacular degeneration).
      ii. Niemann-Pick Disease.
      iii. Gaucher's Disease.
      iv. Metachromatic Leucodystrophy (sulphatide lipidosis).

 b. Disorders of Amino-acid Metabolism.—
  i. Phenylketonuria.
  ii. Tyrosinæmia.
  iii. Homocystinuria.
  iv. Histidinæmia.
  v. Maple Syrup Urine Disease.
  vi. Hartnup Disease.
 c. Disorders of Carbohydrate Metabolism.—
  i. Gargoylism.
  ii. Galactosæmia.
  iii. Hypoglycæmia.
 d. Disorders of Endocrine Metabolism.—
  Cretinism.
 e. Disorders of Mineral and Electrolyte Metabolism.—
  i. Wilson's Disease (hepatolenticular degeneration).
  ii. Diabetes Insipidus.
  iii. Hypomagnesæmia.
 f. Disorders of Nutrition.—
  Malnutrition.

4. **Mental Subnormality associated with Postnatal Brain Disease.—**
 a. Neurofibromatosis.
 b. Sturge-Weber's Syndrome.
 c. Tuberous Sclerosis.
 d. Schilder's Disease.

5. **Mental Subnormality associated with Diseases and Conditions due to Prenatal Factors.—**
 a. Craniostenosis.
 b. Hydrocephalus.
 c. Hypertelorism.
 d. Microcephaly.
 e. Laurence-Moon-Biedl Syndrome.
 f. Ichthyosis.

6. **Mental Subnormality with Chromosomal Abnormalities.—**
 a. Down's Syndrome.
 b. Cat-cry Syndrome. 5ᵗʰ chrom.
 c. Edwards " Trisomy 18.
 d. Patau's " " 13-15
 E. De Lange's .

c. Sex Chromosome Abnormalities.—
   i. Klinefelter's Syndrome.
   ii. Turner's Syndrome.
   iii. Triple-X Syndrome.
   iv. XYY Syndrome.
7. **Mental Subnormality associated with Prematurity.—**
  a. Prematurity.
  b. Kernicterus.
  c. Cerebral Palsy.
8. **Unclassified Mental Subnormality.**

MENTAL SUBNORMALITY FOLLOWING INFECTION

Gastro-enteritis in the Newborn.—In the newborn fluid loss and dehydration in gastro-enteritis may be so severe that brain damage with permanent mental retardation results. Intracranial venous thromboses are usually found in such cases.

Meningitis.—Meningitis is an infection of the coverings of the brain. The common types are pyogenic and tuberculous meningitis.

The onset in pyogenic meningitis is sudden, with headache, increasing irritability, and pyrexia. Projectile vomiting occurs. Muscle rigidity is found with stiffness of the neck. Mental retardation may develop as a direct result of meningitis causing severe brain damage or following the development of hydrocephalus, when inflammatory lesions block the flow of cerebrospinal fluid.

Tuberculous meningitis usually develops insidiously. Irritability alternates with drowsiness. There is loss of appetite with vomiting and constipation. During the terminal stage hyperpyrexia occurs with coma and paralysis. With antituberculous drugs the majority of infants recover from the infection, but damage to the central nervous system and mental retardation are still found in some children.

Congenital Syphilis.—Congenital syphilis is now rare in this country. Infection occurs before birth and is due to the passage of the organism *Treponema pallidum* across the placenta from the mother to the infant. Shortly after birth the infected infant becomes pale and wasted and fails to thrive. A rash is visible on the skin and the nail-beds are infected. There are usually moist lesions on the skin around the mouth, anus, and genitals. A characteristic feature is ' snuffles ' due to infection of the bones of the nose, with nasal obstruction and purulent and blood-stained discharge; collapse of the nasal bridge occurs with the formation of the saddle-nose deformity. When the nervous system is involved, signs of meningeal irritation develop and convulsions and hydrocephalus may occur. Late manifestations of syphilis may appear from 1 to 10 years after birth, with maldevelopment of the teeth, damage to the eyes, spastic paralysis, convulsions, and mental retardation. Thorough antisyphilitic treatment is essential when the diagnosis has been made.

Encephalitis.—Encephalitis is an infection of the brain substance. It may occur following infections with measles, rubella, chicken-pox, mumps, encephalitis lethargica, cytomegalic inclusion disease, and toxoplasmosis. The onset of encephalitis is usually sudden with severe headache and drowsiness, progressing to deep coma. However, the onset can be insidious with a gradually increasing headache, convulsions, or behaviour disorders. In young infants mental retardation, nerve palsies, and behaviour disorders are likely to be severe and permanent.

Congenital Rubella Syndrome.—Rubella (German measles), if contracted within the first 3 months of pregnancy, may cause in the infant mental retardation, deafness, cataract, and heart disease.

Cytomegalic Inclusion Disease.—This virus disease in the mother is usually mild. Infection of the fœtus, however, gives rise to mental retardation and enlargement of the liver and spleen with jaundice. Inclusion bodies can be recognized in tissue cells and in the urine and cerebrospinal fluid.

Toxoplasmosis.—This infection is transmitted to the offspring either late in pregnancy or at the time of birth. It causes mild hydrocephalus or microcephaly, spastic deformities, convulsions, and enlargement of the liver and spleen.

MENTAL SUBNORMALITY FOLLOWING INJURY OR PHYSICAL AGENTS

Pre-eclampsia and Eclampsia.—Pre-eclampsia and eclampsia are conditions which may affect a mother in the last 3 months of pregnancy. There is a rise in the maternal blood-pressure accompanied by severe headache and oedema of the limbs with kidney and liver disorders. Continuous epileptic seizures occur in eclampsia. Stillbirths are common in this condition and live births may show severe brain damage with mental retardation and epileptic attacks later in life.

Excessive Intra-uterine Irradiation.—During the first 3 months of pregnancy irradiation of the uterus may result in microcephaly and mental retardation of ranging degrees of severity.

Birth Injury.—Prematurity, anoxia (an adequate supply of oxygen to the tissues), and difficult labour are important factors in birth injury. Prematurity itself may be a cause of intracranial hæmorrhage and anoxia is common in premature infants. Anoxia due to delay in breathing after birth can cause direct damage to the brain cells and give rise to spastic paralysis and mental retardation. Anoxia can result from the administration of large doses of anæsthetic to the mother, from the inhalation of mucus, or from the constriction of the windpipe (trachea) by the cord being twined tightly around the neck of the infant. Other obstetric difficulties, such as instrumental delivery, precipitate labour, or breech delivery, may produce damage to the brain of the baby.

Rhesus Incompatibility.—About 85 per cent of people carry the Rhesus factor in their red cells ('Rh positive'). The other 15 per cent do not have this factor and are called 'Rh negative'. The condition of rhesus incompatibility occurs when the mother (usually Rh negative) and the fœtus (usually Rh positive) are of different groups. Fœtal blood enters the mother's circulation and stimulates the production of substances called 'antibodies'. Later in pregnancy these antibodies return across the placenta to destroy the fœtal red blood-cells; a condition known as 'hæmolytic disease in the newborn'. Recently it has been discovered that injection of mothers with antibodies obtained from previously immunized mothers prevents the formation of antibodies in a subsequent pregnancy.

Drugs and the Newborn.—Some drugs taken by the mother during pregnancy and by the infant after birth can affect the development of the infant and give rise to mental retardation.

Excessive intake of vitamin D can cause infantile hypercalcæmia. Children so affected become ill shortly after birth with vomiting and constipation. Muscle weakness occurs with thirst and increased output of urine. The blood calcium is raised. Many of these children have elfin faces with low-set ears and prominent epicanthic folds. Heart murmurs are found and the child is usually mentally retarded.

Enzyme systems in the liver of the infant can be affected by excess of vitamin K and by some antibiotics giving rise to jaundice and kernicterus with possible brain damage.

Drugs given to the mother to control endocrine, physical, or emotional disorders can cause fœtal damage. Hypoglycæmia (low blood-sugar) usually occurs in these infants and brain damage may follow.

Cretinism may develop in the child of a mother who has had treatment for hyperthyroidism (oversecretion of the thyroid hormone) during her pregnancy.

Lead Poisoning.—Ingestion of lead by children may lead to mental retardation. Lead may be absorbed from paint, toys, ointments, and cosmetics. The symptoms include loss of appetite, constipation, headache, irritability, delirium, and convulsions.

MENTAL SUBNORMALITY ASSOCIATED WITH DISORDERS OF METABOLISM

Disorders of Lipid Metabolism.—These conditions form a rare group of diffuse and progressive disorders of childhood which have a common feature of progressive mental subnormality. They are storage diseases in which various lipids are deposited in the cells of the central nervous system and the tissues of the body. There is no treatment at present available for these conditions.

Amaurotic Family Idiocy (Cerebromacular Degeneration).— This is a rare condition due to a single recessive gene. There is a deposition of a lipid material within the nerve cells leading to their degeneration. Tay-Sachs disease is the commonest form and is a disease which mostly affects the Jewish race. The child is normal at birth and develops normally until about the end of the third month when spasticity, generalized weakness, and muscle wasting occur. A characteristic feature is that the infant is easily startled by loud noises. There is progressive loss of vision leading to complete blindness. A 'cherry-red' spot is found in the macula of the retina. Death usually takes place within 2 years of the onset of the disease. The other types of amaurotic family idiocy have similar presentations but develop later in life.

Niemann-Pick Disease.—The onset of this disease is during infancy and death often occurs before the second year. The disease is characterized by mental deterioration and retardation with the physical features of wasting, profuse sweating, and yellowish pigmentation of the skin. The liver, spleen, and lymph-glands are enlarged. There is loss of vision and hearing. A cherry-red spot at the macula as seen in amaurotic family idiocy is often observed.

Gaucher's Disease.—This is an uncommon disorder of lipid metabolism. The cells of the reticulo-endothelial system contain deposits of lipid material which lead to an enlargement of the liver, spleen, and lymph-nodes. In cases with an acute onset the brain may be involved resulting in mental subnormality. The disease is due to an autosomal recessive gene.

Metachromatic Leucodystrophy (Sulphatide Lipidosis).—Metachromatic leucodystrophy is a familial disease found in late infancy which causes severe brain damage. The child appears normal for the first year or two but then progressive muscular weakness and incoordination develop. Death usually occurs between the third and sixth years in this disease. Sulphatides accumulate in the brain and kidney and the accumulation of these substances interferes with normal brain function. A screening test using fresh urine is now available.

Disorders of Amino-acid Metabolism.—

Phenylketonuria.—Phenylketonuria is an inborn error of metabolism commonly accompanied by severe mental defect. The basic fault is deficiency of the enzyme normally responsible for converting the amino-acid phenylalanine to the amino-acid tyrosine so that phenylalanine, phenylpyruvic acid, and their toxic products accumulate in the blood and are subsequently excreted in the urine.

The patient affected with phenylketonuria is nearly always fair haired with light blue eyes. The skin is fair, soft, smooth, and fine in texture. There is frequent occurrence of eczema and there is often cyanosis of the hands and feet due to poor circulation. The patient is dwarfed and a slightly reduced head circumference is not uncommon. The gait is stiff, short-stepped, and on a broad base. The incisor teeth are widely spaced. Some phenylketonurics show stiffness in their limbs. Epilepsy occurs in the majority of patients. Repetitive finger movements are seen in the lower-grade patient.

Mass screening for amino-acid abnormalities in the newborn is at present proceeding in many centres. The Guthrie test which is a bacteriological method detects raised levels of phenylalanine. When the plasma phenylalanine rises above 4 mg. per cent a diagnosis of phenylketonuria is considered. Other methods using chromatography are being developed and these methods, unlike the Guthrie test, can detect the other amino-acid abnormalities present at birth.

Phenylketonuria, when detected at birth, is treated with a low phenylalanine diet and the onset of mental defect is prevented.

Tyrosinæmia.—There are two types of disorder of tyrosine metabolism in the newborn. Transient tyrosinæmia is the condition in which there are elevated plasma tyrosine levels which decrease as the child gets older. Usually the only reason why these infants come to notice is that a positive test for tyrosinæmia is found when testing for phenylketonuria in the newborn. Infants with transient tyrosinæmia are physically normal in all respects. The more permanent disorder of tyrosine metabolism is tyrosinosis. Within a few days of birth children affected with this disorder develop severe vomiting and diarrhœa. They fail to thrive and progressive liver failure and severe kidney damage occur. Children who survive suffer from mental retardation. Dietary treatment is, however, available for this condition.

Homocystinuria.—Homocystinuria is an inborn error of sulphur amino-acid metabolism. The amino-acid methionine is increased in the blood and the amino-acid homocystine appears in the urine. In homocystinuria the patient has certain signs and symptoms, some mild and some severe. These symptoms are dislocated lenses, fine, sparse hair, convulsions, flush of the cheek, knock knees, and mental retardation.

Affected patients can be detected by a simple urine test and dietary treatment is now being tried.

Histidinæmia.—Histidinæmia is caused by an enzyme defect in the metabolism of the amino-acid histidine. Urine from these patients shows a positive test with Phenistix, but phenylpyruvic acid is not present in the urine. Affected patients show a speech defect and some are mentally retarded.

Maple Syrup Urine Disease.—This condition is so called because of its sweet-smelling urine which is said to resemble the smell of maple syrup. The blood and urine contain abnormal amounts of the amino-acids valine, leucine, and isoleucine. single autosomal recessive gene.

Affected patients show clinical symptoms shortly after birth. There is difficulty in feeding and the respiration is irregular. Stiffness of the limbs is found. Rapid physical deterioration occurs and the infants die within a few weeks or months.

The condition can be treated with a diet which is deficient in the amino-acids valine, leucine, and isoleucine.

Hartnup Disease.—This condition resembles pellagra and is an abnormality in the metabolism of the amino-acid tryptophane leading to a pellagra-like skin rash, temporary cerebellar ataxia, constant amino-aciduria, and the excretion of large amounts of indole substances. Some of the patients affected have been mental defectives.

Disorders of Carbohydrate Metabolism.—

Gargoylism.—Gargoylism is a rare type of mental subnormality caused by a single recessive gene and is characterized by the deposition of mucopolysaccharide in the tissue cells of the brain, liver, heart and lungs, and spleen. There are two main types of gargoylism. In the first type both males and females are equally affected and cousin marriages are frequent precipitating factors. Clouding of the cornea and dwarfism occur. The second type is sex-linked. Only males are affected. Corneal clouding does not occur and only one-third of patients are small of stature. Half of the patients affected are deaf, however.

The name 'gargoylism' is evocative and describes the strange appearance of the affected patients. The head is enlarged and the forehead protrudes. The eyebrows are bushy and the nose is saddle-shaped. The abdomen is protuberant and there is usually an umbilical hernia. Considerable enlargement of the liver and spleen is found. The degree of mental subnormality varies. There is no treatment at present for gargoylism.

Galactosæmia.—This is a rare congenital and familial disorder in which the sugar galactose is not converted into glucose in the normal manner due to an enzyme defect. It is caused by a single autosomal recessive gene. The infant with this condition appears normal at birth but after a few days' milk feeding loses his appetite and has persistent vomiting. In severe cases death occurs from malnutrition. Those who survive are at 3 months of age undernourished and small in stature. Mental retardation and cataracts occur. Examination of the urine shows a constant presence of the sugar galactose and an increased excretion of amino-acids and protein. If diagnosed shortly after birth, the signs and symptoms disappear after the removal of milk and milk products from the diet.

Hypoglycæmia in the Newborn.—Hypoglycæmia or low blood-sugar in the newborn has many causes. It is found in premature infants and in twins and is more common in male than in female births. It can be familial and mothers with diabetes mellitus and toxæmia of pregnancy may give birth to infants with hypoglycæmia.

Infants with hypoglycæmia are pale and reluctant to feed. They are irritable and the infant is said to be 'jittery'. Convulsions may occur. Treatment is by correction of the cause, but if the hypoglycæmia in the infant is severe prolonged brain damage will occur.

Disorders of Endocrine Metabolism.—

Cretinism.—The condition of cretinism is due to a defect of the thyroid gland resulting from various enzyme disturbances. The early signs of the disease are feeding difficulties, noisy respiration, constipation, and jaundice. The child's growth is retarded. He is apathetic and he does not readily smile or laugh and is slow to suck. The tongue becomes large and protrudes as the condition progresses. The skin becomes yellowish, loose, and wrinkled, with marked puffiness of the eyes and thickening of the eyelids, nostrils, lips, hands, feet, and back of the neck. Prominence of the abdomen with an umbilical hernia is common. The hair on the scalp and eyebrows is often very scanty. The child has a peculiar hoarse cry. With the lapse of time the child makes little attempt to sit up, stand, or walk. Speech may not appear until 7 or 8 years of age. The characteristic features of untreated cases are severe mental defect, dwarfed stature, bowed small legs, and stumpy hands and feet. The eyes are set widely apart and the lips are pouting. The nose is broad and flattened. Puberty is usually late in appearing and the external genitals remain infantile.

In the majority of cases thyroid treatment is effective if the diagnosis is made at an early stage.

Disorders of Mineral and Electrolyte Metabolism.—

Wilson's Disease (Hepatolenticular Degeneration).—This condition is accompanied by a decrease of copper and the copper-containing protein cæruloplasmin in the serum. The symptoms occur after the age of 10 years in a child who has previously been mentally normal. Involuntary choreiform movements with tremor develop with progressive difficulty in articulation and swallowing. Rigidity of the muscles of limbs, trunk, and face occur resulting in contractures of the limbs and muscle wasting. A smoky brownish ring (Kayser-Fleischer ring) forms at the outer margin of the cornea. There is progressive mental and physical deterioration. Treatment with penicillamine by increasing copper excretion in the urine is helpful in some cases of Wilson's disease.

Diabetes Insipidus.—This condition is due to a sex-linked recessive gene. It affects males who are unable to control the passage of water from the blood to the kidneys. In early infancy the child develops an excessive thirst and passes large amounts of urine. He becomes dehydrated and may run erratic fevers. This condition is prevented by continuous large intakes of water.

Hypomagnesæmia.—Infants born to mothers who are suffering from magnesium deficiency may develop convulsions in the neonatal period. Hypomagnesæmia also develops when severe malnutrition is complicated by chronic diarrhœa. These convulsions, especially if complicated by dehydration and malnutrition, are liable to cause permanent brain damage. Adequate replacement of the deficient magnesium rapidly relieves the condition.

Disorders of Nutrition in the Infant.—

Malnutrition.—Malnutrition is now recognized as one of the postnatal causes of mental retardation. Severe malnutrition during the first 2 years of life, when brain growth is most active, may result in permanent reduction of brain size with mental defect.

MENTAL SUBNORMALITY ASSOCIATED WITH POSTNATAL BRAIN DISEASE

Neurofibromatosis.—This is a hereditary disease characterized by pigmentation of the skin and tumours of the nerve trunks and skin. Tumours may occur within the skull and give rise to mental symptoms and epilepsy.

Sturge-Weber's Syndrome.—The causative factor is unknown. The condition is characterized by nævus of the face on one side only, meningeal angioma, possible calcification of the cerebral cortex, epilepsy, hemiplegia, and severe subnormality.

Tuberous Sclerosis.—This condition is due to a single dominant gene. The three cardinal symptoms of this condition are mental subnormality, epilepsy, and adenoma sebaceum.

Most of these patients are severely subnormal and, as they grow, they undergo progressive mental deterioration and most die before reaching maturity. Epileptic fits occur from the first year of life and continue with increased severity. Status epilepticus is the commonest cause of death. Adenoma sebaceum (butterfly rash) is a rash arranged symmetrically on both cheeks and involving the nose. It is due to an overgrowth of the sebaceous glands of the skin. Post-mortem examination often reveals tumours of various internal organs and of the brain.

Schilder's Disease.—This condition is due to a single recessive gene. Defective synthesis of myelin is associated with axon degeneration and neuronal overgrowth.

The disease usually makes its appearance in childhood or adolescence. The clinical features, which vary considerably, consist of progressive failure of vision and hearing, spastic paralysis, convulsive attacks, muscular incoordination of the limbs, and tonic and clonic spasms. Difficulty in swallowing and speaking may be experienced by some patients. The mental impairment is progressive.

MENTAL SUBNORMALITY ASSOCIATED WITH DISEASES AND CONDITIONS DUE TO PRENATAL FACTORS

Craniostenosis.—Although the cause of this condition is unknown it is thought possible to be due to a dominant gene. Not all patients are mentally subnormal. The condition is characterized by an elongated skull, protuberant eyes, and a high narrow palate. There may be developmental abnormalities of the limbs, such as rudimentary fingers and thumb.

Hydrocephalus.—Hydrocephalus, 'water on the brain', refers to an increased volume of cerebrospinal fluid within the skull. The excess cerebrospinal fluid may be within the ventricles or in the subarachnoid space. In the infant the head expands to accommodate the excessive fluid; as a result the circumference of the head may increase to as much as 36 inches (90 cm.)—the normal average adult circumference being 22 inches (55 cm.).

The hydrocephalus may be primary or secondary. Primary hydrocephalus results from developmental abnormalities

4

causing excessive secretion of the cerebrospinal fluid and a low or absent absorption of the secreted fluids. Secondary hydrocephalus is caused by lesions within the system of ducts which drain away the cerebrospinal fluid. Blockage of these ducts causes an obstruction to the flow of fluids. Those commonly affected are the aqueduct of Sylvius and the foramina of Luschka and Magendie.

The hydrocephalus may be active, producing progressive deterioration. The patient will suffer from blindness, deafness, and convulsions, be severely wasted, bedridden, and paralysed. Death usually takes place very early in life. In patients who survive the condition is only slowly progressive and is often arrested, leaving the patient with varying degrees of mental and physical disability. The majority of hydrocephalics are quiet, affectionate, tractable, obedient, and willing. Physically they tend to be undersized with some muscular weakness and spasticity which affect the legs causing their movements to be clumsy and incoordinated.

Hypertelorism.—Hypertelorism is a rare form of mental subnormality. There is abnormal development of the sphenoid bone of the skull and this thrusts the brow forward, separating the nasal bones more widely than normal. The distance between the eyes is increased and in extreme cases the eyes tend to appear on the side of the face. Hare-lip and cleft palate may occur. The patient is usually subnormal.

Microcephaly.—Microcephaly is the name applied to mentally subnormal persons whose cranium on completion of development is less than 17 inches (42·5 cm.) in circumference. This condition is due to a single recessive gene which determines the inability of the brain to develop to its normal size.

The head is reduced in size so that a relatively normal nose and chin and large ears contrast with the receding forehead and flattened back of head. There is overlapping of the sutures of the skull and thick ridges of bone can be felt. The scalp is sometimes loose and wrinkled longitudinally as though too big for the skull. The majority of affected patients are within the severely subnormal range although some may be subnormal.

Microcephaly is not always a specific disease. It is often a feature of other clinical types of mental subnormality. **Laurence-Moon-Biedl-Syndrome.**—This is a very rare condition which is thought to be due to a recessive gene defect and is characterized by obesity, hypogenitalism, extra fingers and toes, eye defects which include pigmentary degeneration of the retina, nystagmus, optic atrophy, poor night vision and progressive visual defect, and severe subnormality. **Ichthyosis.**—Ichthyosis is a congenital skin disease characterized by scaling and hyperkeratosis and is a common complaint in the general population. Several genes may cause it. The most frequent is an autosomal dominant. There are two syndromes associated with mental deficiency of which ichthyosis is an essential part. The Sjogren-Larsson syndrome is characterized by spastic diplegia, ichthyosis, and mental subnormality. Rud's syndrome is characterized by ichthyosis, sexual infantilism, epilepsy, and mild subnormality.

MENTAL SUBNORMALITY WITH CHROMOSOMAL ABNORMALITIES

A human being originates in the union of two sex cells (gametes), the ovum and the spermatozoa, and is built up of single units called ' cells '. Each cell is composed of a cell membrane which surrounds the complex cell structures which include the cytoplasm (a substance surrounding the nucleus) and the nucleus itself—a compact object containing the hereditary material, chromosomes, in the form of strands of desoxyribonucleic acid, a substance commonly known as DNA.

DNA is the main compound of the chromosomes but they also contain ribonucleic acid (RNA) and protein. Other indefinite structures are present also and are called ' genes '. Genes are ' blueprints ' for the development of the individual. The position of the gene on the chromosome is called its ' locus'. Genes occasionally change their character giving rise to new genes. This process is called ' mutation '.

Some genes are capable of producing dominant and recessive traits. A dominant trait is the result of a defective gene in one or both parents and has the following characteristics :—

1. Every affected person has an affected parent.

2. The affected person is easily distinguishable.

3. In every affected family one-half of the children will be affected.

Recessive traits are caused by the occurrence of two similarly defective genes, one from each parent, and have the following characteristics :—

1. The parents are carriers of the defective gene.

2. The parents are normal with respect to the defective trait.

3. In every affected family one-quarter of the children will be affected ; one-half will be carriers of the defective trait.

Genes may be linked to sex and whether an individual develops normally or abnormally may depend upon the sex of the individual.

The hereditary material in the cells of man is divided into 46 sections of varying lengths making 23 pairs of different chromosomes. When the genes of a pair of like chromosomes (' homologous ') contain comparable sets of loci then they are said to be ' homozygous '. If they do not agree they are ' heterozygous '.

These arrangements apply to 22 pairs of chromosomes (the ' autosomes ') ; the sex chromosomes in the male differ, one being an X and the other Y, whilst in the female they are a homologous pair XX.

Transmission of the hereditary material from one generation to another takes place through the germ cells, the spermatozoa in the male and the ova in the female. These cells unlike the other cells of the body have each only one-half the normal complement of chromosomes, 23 in number. When fertilization takes place the sperm and the ovum unite together to form a new individual and this is called the ' zygote '. Thus each individual has received one-half of his chromosomes from each of his parents.

Down's Syndrome (Mongolism).—Although Langdon Down first described mongolism a hundred years ago it is only during the past few years that it has been recognized that the condition is the result of a chromosome abnormality. It is now known that Down's syndrome is caused by the presence of an extra chromosome in pair 21. Three types of Down's syndrome occur :—

PLATE I

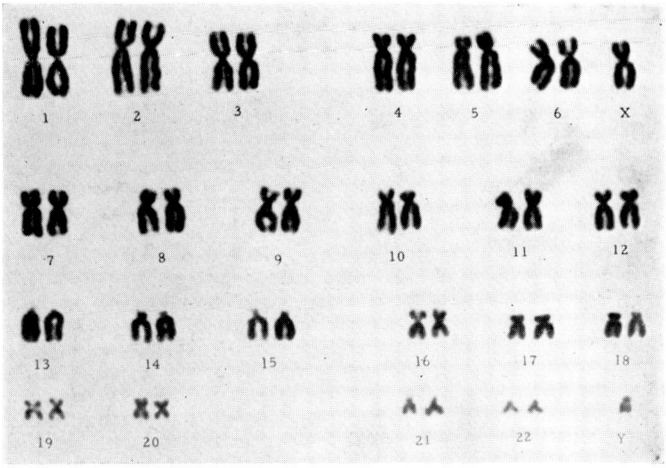

A

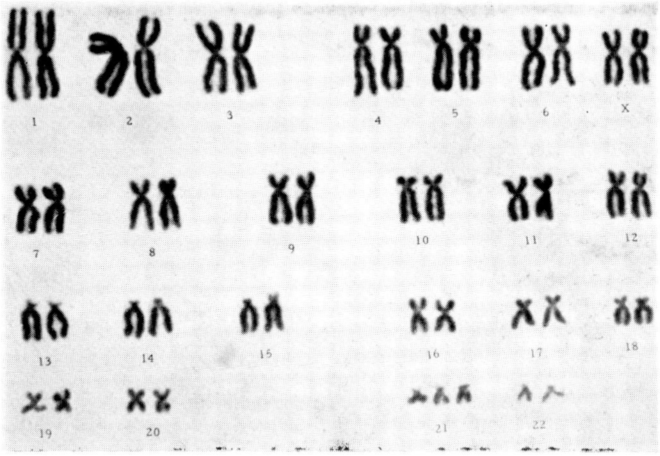

B

A, A photograph of human (male) chromosomes; B, A photograph of human (female) chromosomes, illustrating a case of trisomy of 21 (female mongol).

<u>Dominant Gene</u>
Huntington's Chorea.
Tuberous Sclerosis, (Epiloia.)
Acrocephaly.
Marfan's Syn.

a. Regular : The chromosome count is 47 instead of the 'ormal 46, the extra chromosome being one of the smaller 1romosomes.

b. Translocation : The chromosome count remains at 46, 1e extra small chromosome has become attached to another 1romosome making the chromosomal count appear normal.

c. Mosaic : The chromosome count is 46 in some cells and 7 in other cells.

Down's syndrome accounts for 10 per cent of all patients 1dmitted to mental deficiency hospitals. The incidence in the general population is 1 per 700 births. Cases tend to be born at the end of large families and the frequency is related closely to the age of the mother ; the risk of giving birth to a child with Down's syndrome rises with the age of the mother. More than one case can occur in a family. Other chromosomal abnormalities such as Klinefelter's syndrome, Triple-X syndrome, and Turner's syndrome have been found in association with Down's syndrome. Acute leukaemia is more prevalent in Down's syndrome than in the general population.

Principal Features of Down's Syndrome.—These are stunted growth, a small round head with flat face and occiput, a florid complexion, and obliquely set eyelids, with upper lids having an extra fold at the inner margin (epicanthic fold). There may be eye defects such as squint, nystagmus, and cataract. The ears are small and do not possess the natural folds. The nose is stubby and depressed at the bridge ; the tongue in most cases is large and flabby with well-defined fissures. The hair is dry and scanty. The hands are broad and clumsy-looking and have a curious 'boggy' feeling. The little finger is curved and ends midway between the last and middle interphalangeal joints of the third finger. The palm creases are abnormal ; a single transverse crease often runs across the palm of the hand. The feet are marked by a large cleft between the first and second toes and often a crease runs from this cleft down the sole of the foot. Supernumerary toes and webbing of the toes are seen occasionally. The abdomen is protuberant and umbilical hernia is common. The joints have abnormal range of movement due to laxity of the ligaments and hypotonus of the muscles. The circulation is usually poor, the extremities being blue and cold and susceptible to chilblains.   Mongols are usually mouth breathers and are prone to respiratory infections.

Mentally the mongol has a happy and cheerful disposition. He is good tempered, affectionate, and easily amused.   He is a good mimic, has a fondness for dancing and music, and has a good sense of rhythm.

Cat-cry Syndrome.—In this condition affected infants are severely mentally retarded and have a characteristic mewing cry from which the syndrome gets its name.   In appearance they are obviously abnormal with small heads, wide-spaced eyes, epicanthic folds, abnormalities of the ears and mouth, and eyes slanting downwards.   The condition is due to partial deletion of the short arm of chromosome No. 4 or 5.

Sex Chromosome Abnormalities.—The true genetic sex of an individual can be determined by obtaining preparations from the cells lining the inside of the mouth (buccal smear) and examining them for the presence of the sex chromatin body.   This body is found in the nuclei of females (chromatin positive) and is absent in males (chromatin negative).

The sex chromosome abnormalities are :— *haemophilia, allbine and colour blind*

Klinefelter's Syndrome.—The patient is a male whose sex chromatin is positive.   The sex chromosome constitution is XXY and the total chromosome count is 47.   After puberty, patients with this constitution present with sterility and have small testicles.   The breasts may be feminine in appearance and eunuchoidism may occur.   The degree of mental subnormality varies but is usually mild.   The frequency of the condition is 1 per 750 births.

Turner's Syndrome.—The patient is female with absent sex chromatin.   The cells have only a single X chromosome and the total chromosome count is 45.   The patients are dwarfed and congenital abnormalities are found, particularly webbing of the neck.   At puberty secondary sexual development is absent due to lack of ovarian tissue and hormones.   The degree of mental subnormality is usually mild.   The frequency of this condition is 1 per 3000 births.

Triple-X Syndrome.—The patient is female and there are no abnormal physical characteristics. The sex chromosome constitution is XXX and the total chromosome count is 47. The tissue cells are chromatin positive and some cells contain two sex chromatin bodies. The frequency of this condition is 1 per 750 births.

XYY Syndrome.—These patients are of interest as the majority of them have been diagnosed in the maximum security mental hospitals. They are unusually tall, over 6 feet in height, with a tendency towards aggression and violence. As in Klinefelter's syndrome there is some reduction in intelligence.

MENTAL SUBNORMALITY ASSOCIATED WITH PREMATURITY

Prematurity.—By definition any infant weighing 2500 g. ($5\frac{1}{2}$ lb.) or less at birth is premature ; 5–10 per cent of all births are in this category. Premature infants are particularly liable to develop severe respiratory distress at birth and this is associated with a higher mortality-rate. Infants with a birth weight less than 1500 g. show an association between respiratory distress and the development of mental retardation and neurological abnormalities. Prematurity may be found in association with maternal toxæmia, congenital anomalies, and multiple pregnancy. Premature children also have a liability to kernicterus and also hypoglycæmia which may lead to mental retardation.

Kernicterus.—Kernicterus or jaundice of the newborn with brain damage occurs in prematurity, infantile malnutrition, and when some drugs are given to the infant or to the mother. Sepsis and congenital cirrhosis of the liver may also be factors. Kernicterus may also occur in hæmolytic disease of the newborn especially when there is Rhesus antibody incompatibility. The affected infant may be obviously jaundiced at birth or becomes jaundiced a few days later. The infant is severely ill and fails to thrive properly. There is respiratory distress and death may occur at this stage in respiratory failure. The liver and spleen are enlarged. Cyanotic attacks occur and in some cases severe anæmia

results from hæmolysis. With recovery, athetoid movements may be noted as early as 6 months of age. Motor
development is poor, high-tone deafness is frequent, disorders of balance and epilepsy may occur during early childhood.

Cerebral Palsy.—Cerebral palsy is a permanent disorder
of movement and posture, due to a non-progressive defect
of the brain occurring in early life. The incidence of cerebral
palsy is about 2 per 1000. Mental retardation and cerebral
palsy are commonly found together, approximately half of
the children affected are of subnormal intelligence. Cerebral
palsy may be found in association with prematurity, anoxia,
multiple pregnancies, kernicterus, and prenatal and postnatal
infections.

UNCLASSIFIED MENTAL SUBNORMALITY

Unclassified mental retardation is applied to those cases
in which there is no evidence of structural or biochemical
abnormality. Approximately 65 per cent of all cases of
mental retardation still have to be placed in this unknown
group. The degree of mental retardation varies from the
severely subnormal to the subnormal.

Unclassified mental defect can be divided into two groups.
In the genetic group heredity plays an important part.
Children can show different levels of intellectual development
from their parents, and parents who are themselves below
average in intelligence may produce children who are above
or below their own measured intelligence. Many of the
higher grades of unclassified mental defect belong to the
genetic group. The subcultural group is more complex and
comprises a mixture of genetic and environmental factors.
Below-average parents and adverse home circumstances and
upbringing give rise to this subcultural group of mental
defectives with intelligence quotients in the range of 50 to 70.
Social changes will eventually bring about a reduction in
this type of mental defect.

CHAPTER IV

PHYSICAL CONCOMITANTS

THERE are many associated conditions with mental subnormality which in themselves create problems of communication, training, and care. To name a few there are :—

1. Epilepsy.
2. Hyperkinetic Behaviour.
3. Cerebral Palsy.
4. Autism.
5. Speechlessness (mutism).
6. Deafness.
7. Blindness.
8. Physical Handicaps.

Each one places its own particular limitations on a child's progress.

The nurse is not alone in dealing with and conquering these complex problems, but she must be prepared to work with and co-operate with specialists from other fields without feeling that they are impostors trespassing on her preserves and posing as a threat to her professional status. The nurse should try to realize that patients are often in need of types of specialist treatment which she is not always in a position to give without the advice and guidance from a person qualified in that particular skill. To be a trained nurse does not mean that we are qualified to practise every speciality ; it does mean, however, that the nurse can, as a result of her comprehensive training, supplement the service given by the specially trained personnel such as the special school teacher, speech therapist, occupational therapist, physiotherapist, and skilled craftsman. If the nurse will accept the team principle the rest will come easily. In accepting these other professional people as those who have something to offer the patient, the nurse is not destroying herself, but giving herself the time to practise the skill for which she was trained, the skill of psychiatric nursing. To become too involved in other professional activities will only act as a barrier to the nurse's practice of psychiatric nursing.

EPILEPSY

An acceptable definition of epilepsy is ' a sudden abnormal electrical discharge in the grey matter of the brain which develops suddenly, ceases spontaneously, and exhibits a tendency to recurrence '.

Epilepsy is generally regarded as a symptom of some underlying cause. In some cases a local lesion of the brain plays a part in causation, in others hereditary predisposition seems to be the important factor. Certain chemical changes in the body greatly increase the tendency towards fits or may be responsible for their actual precipitation, such as hypoglycæmia (a diminished blood-sugar), alkalosis, a change in the reaction of the blood towards alkalinity, and uræmia, when the composition of the blood is abnormal owing to defective action of the kidneys, and in some other toxic states.

The nature of the attacks depends upon the area of the brain being affected. The prevalence of epilepsy among the mentally subnormal patients in hospital is fairly high, ranging between 10 and 25 per cent. It is more prevalent amongst the lower level of the mentally subnormal. This may be because of the severe brain damage often found in the severely subnormal patient.

BACKGROUND TO THE INCIDENCE OF EPILEPTIC ATTACKS

The following information will be required by the doctor of a patient suffering from epilepsy :—

1. When did the fits first occur?
2. Was the fit precipitated by an accident or associated with an acute illness?
3. How soon are the fits followed by a second?
4. What is the usual interval between attacks?
5. Are they increasing in frequency?

6. Do the attacks occur in bouts?

7. Has the patient had a series of attacks without recovering consciousness?

8. Do the attacks occur at any special time of the day?

9. Do they occur only by day or only by night?

10. In the case of a woman are they related to the menstrual periods?

11. Is any factor known to precipitate the attacks?

12. Does the patient have any warning? If so, what, and how long does it precede the attack?

13. How does an attack begin? Is its onset local or general, gradual or sudden?

14. Is consciousness lost?

15. Do convulsive movements occur in the attacks? If so, are they symmetrical or asymmetrical?

16. Has the patient injured himself in an attack?

17. Does he bite his tongue and pass urine?

18. How long do the attacks last?

19. What is his condition afterwards?

20. Are the attacks followed by headache, sleepiness, paralysis, or mental disturbance, such as automatism?

21. What treatment has he had and how has he responded to it?

22. Has he at any time suffered from head injury?

23. If the attacks did not begin in infancy, did he suffer from infantile convulsions?

There are several forms of epileptic attack. The main types affecting the mentally subnormal patient in a greater or lesser degree are : (1) Major epilepsy (grand mal) ; (2) Minor epilepsy (petit mal) ; (3) Psychomotor attacks ; (4) Jacksonian epilepsy ; (5) Tonic epilepsy ; (6) Pyknolepsy ; (7) Myoclonus.

THE SYMPTOMS OF EPILEPSY

Major Epilepsy (Grand Mal).—

Preconvulsive Symptoms.—Frequently patients exhibit symptoms for hours or even a day preceding a fit. These symptoms include mental changes, such as irritability and depression, abnormal feelings referred to the head, giddiness, and sudden myoclonic twitches.

Precipitating Factors.—Usually these are absent, but occasionally excitement, excessive noise, and constipation may be present. ' Flicker ' excitations, such as the flicker of the television screen, neon signs, electric lights, and the movement of light through railings, may be precipitating factors.

The Aura.—The aura, or warning, is an experience which usually precedes the onset of unconsciousness. It may be classified as follows : (1) Somatic sensibility ; (2) Visceral sensibility ; (3) Confusion and feeling of detachment ; (4) Special sensations : olfactory, visual, aural, and gustatory disturbances.

It is sometimes noticed that the fit begins with movements of the body. For example, turning the head to one side and flexion of the upper limb ; sometimes the whole body is rotated to one side.

The Onset.—The patient loses consciousness and falls to the ground, often injuring himself, and occasionally gives out a harsh scream due to the forcible expiration of air through the partly closed vocal cords.

The Tonic Spasm of the Muscles.—The muscles of the body go into tonic contractions. This is usually symmetrical on the two sides of the body, causing a state of extension and slight arching of the back. Due to the spasm of the trunk muscles and respiratory muscles, respiration is arrested. The duration of the tonic spasm may extend from a few seconds to half a minute. Progressive cyanosis results from the arrest of respirations.

The Clonic Phase.—The sustained tonic contractions of the muscles give place to sharp, short, interrupted jerks. The tongue may be bitten ; foaming at the mouth may occur. Incontinence of urine very often occurs, but incontinence of fæces is less common.

Towards the end of the clonic stage the muscle jerks become less frequent and finally cease.

The Exhaustion Phase.—The patient remains unconscious for a variable time, extending from a few minutes to half an hour, and on recovery from unconsciousness he often sleeps for several hours.

Headache and confusion are common after an attack.

Sometimes the epileptic fit passes into a hysterical attack, but usually the patient is mentally normal after an attack.

Minor Epilepsy (Petit Mal).—' Minor epilepsy ' is a term applied to a slight epileptic attack and has many manifestations. The slightest form of attack may only occur as a sensation which consists of a disturbance of consciousness, often similar to the aura of a major attack and sometimes associated with giddiness; in a sensation, consciousness may not be completely lost.   In a more severe attack, loss of consciousness is complete, though the patient does not fall, but remains standing owing to the motor and postural function of the brain being little affected.   He looks a little dazed and the eyes have a staring appearance.   After a few seconds he recovers and may continue what he was doing before the attack.

In the most severe petit mal attack the patient loses consciousness and usually falls to the ground, or he may have rigidity of the muscles.

Pallor usually accompanies petit mal and the patient may be incontinent of urine.   Occasionally ' epileptic fugue ' follows as a complication, which is characterized by a loss of memory for any antisocial acts committed.

Psychomotor Attacks.—The patient does not lose consciousness but he does become confused, is often anxious and negativistic, and carries out movements of a highly organized but semi-automatic character.   The attack lasts from a few seconds to a minute or two.

Jacksonian Epilepsy.—These attacks are usually symptoms of organic disease of the brain. The attack usually begins with clonic spasm of a small area of the opposite side to the brain lesion, either in the thumb, index finger, great toe, or angle of the mouth. As the convulsions become more severe they spread to the other limb of the same side of the body, then to the face, and finally they become bilateral. Consciousness is never lost ; this is usually diagnostic. The patient is always aware of factors in his environment. His memory is unaffected by an attack.

Tonic Epilepsy.—In the usual form of tonic epilepsy the head is extended, the upper limbs are thrown out in front of the patient extended at the elbows, the lower limbs are extended, and oculogyric crises are common. This type of fit is usually the result of organic disease of the brain.

Pyknolepsy.—This is a form of epilepsy characterized by very frequent attacks of petit mal. It occurs in children and the patient may have as many as 100 attacks in a day. The onset is usually sudden and ends spontaneously. Treatment does not appear to have any effect on the attacks.

Myoclonus Epilepsy.—A familial condition occurring in several children in the same family.

The onset of the symptoms occurs as a rule between the ages of 6 and 16 years and is characterized by generalized epileptiform attacks with loss of consciousness occurring at night.

As the condition progresses the characteristic myoclonic contractions develop. These are shock-like muscular contractions affecting the muscles of the face, trunk, and upper and lower limbs. They disappear during sleep and are made worse by emotional excitement. Myoclonus also affects the lips and tongue, interfering with speech and swallowing. The usual treatment for epilepsy will control the generalized epilepsy but has less influence upon the myoclonus.

Status Epilepticus.—It is not uncommon for one fit to follow another within a few hours or days. Occasionally there occurs a constant succession of attacks extending over many hours and with such rapidity that the patient appears never to come out of the one fit. This condition is often followed by fatal results and demands urgent medical attention.

THE NURSING ASPECTS OF EPILEPSY

Patients suffering from epilepsy very often have little else in common with other patients also suffering from epilepsy. It is therefore impractical to nurse them all in the same ward. Some are so disturbed as to need constant supervision, while others are quiet and tractable and require only casual supervision ; very often they are the most efficient and most reliable workers.

The epileptic patient should share as fully as possible in the life of the hospital. If his fits are well under control there should be little difficulty in finding a suitable ward and suitable occupation and recreation. It should always be remembered that he will need supervision and should not be allowed to work in any place where a fit might endanger his life or the lives of others.

OBSERVATION

The nurse's observation will be of invaluable assistance to the doctor in assessing the patient's medical requirements. At first the nurse may be upset and excited and therefore too emotionally involved to be able to give a very accurate report. After the first experience she will be able to keep calm and her observation should improve. As soon as the nurse has observed a patient having a fit and carried out all the essential nursing care she should write down all her observations which should include :—

1. Duration of fit.
2. Duration of each stage.
3. The frequency of the fits.
4. Was the patient upset prior to the fit?
5. Any other suspected precipitating factors.
6. Was the nurse aware of an impending attack? If so, in what form did this awareness appear?
7. To know the direction of the fall will have valuable significance to the doctor.
8. Also of value are the observation of the muscle tone during the fit, observing whether the tonic stage is unilateral or bilateral; whether it starts simultaneously throughout the whole body, or on which side or which part of the body it first appears. The order in which the various parts of the body are affected may be important.
9. As soon as the attack has ceased, the pulse and respiration are recorded and the colour is noted.
10. A report should also be made on whether the patient has bitten his tongue and if he was incontinent.
11. After the fit a record of the duration and the depth of sleep should be made.
12. On return to consciousness any complaints of headache, vomiting, or signs of confusion either in speech or action, and their duration, should be recorded.

THE TREATMENT OF EPILEPSY

The treatment of an epileptic patient may be put under two headings : (1) Medical treatment ; (2) Nursing treatment.

MEDICAL TREATMENT

Two advances in recent years have radically altered the treatment of epilepsy :—

1. **Electro-encephalograph.**—The use of this as a routine procedure has enabled the diagnosis of epilepsy to be made with greater precision and has helped to differentiate the various types.

2. **Drugs.**—The discovery of drugs with anticonvulsant activity which have very little sedative effect.

Resulting from these advances the doctors are able to make a more precise assessment of a patient's epileptic condition and of his treatment requirements.

It is well known that drugs which benefit one form of epilepsy may be of no value in another form of the disease ; they may even aggravate it.

Before the doctor administers any drug to an epileptic patient he will have investigated the nature of the epileptic seizure, which will include encephalography. A study of the individual patient's needs will be made. The administration of anticonvulsant drugs is usually related to the timing and frequency of the seizures. For example, a patient who has his attacks mainly at night or on waking will take his dose at night and will require little or no medication throughout the day ; women who have premenstrual attacks may require anticonvulsants only during the week before the period.

The doctor will begin a patient's treatment using drugs he is familiar with and he will gradually increase the dose until the seizures are controlled or until side-effects or symptoms of toxicity appear.

Phenobarbitone will usually be the first choice. It is relatively free from toxic effects though it does have hypnotic effects.

Phenytoin is also a drug of first choice in major epilepsy, though the incidence of side-effects and toxicity is greater. In combination phenobarbitone and phenytoin have an additive effect and are often successful when singly they have failed. For petit mal troxidene or ethosuximide are the first-choice drugs with acetazolamide as a useful alternative or as an additional preparation. Phenobarbitone often makes the patient with petit mal worse ; when drowsiness is a problem a small dose of amphetamine is often helpful. Psychomotor epilepsy is the most difficult to control. Primidone is frequently the drug of first choice, though phenytoin and succinimide are often used. In ' status epilepticus ' an intramuscular injection of 8–10 ml. paraldehyde may be given, followed by 5 ml. every 30 minutes as required.

NURSING TREATMENT

The nursing treatment of an epileptic patient may be divided into three stages : (1) Before the fit ; (2) During the fit ; (3) After the fit.

1. Before the Fit.—The epileptic patient should as far as possible live a normal life. Children should attend school and be subject to ordinary discipline. Adults should carry on an occupation geared to their level of work ability. Occupations involving working at heights, near machinery, or driving should not be undertaken.

It is impossible to guard an epileptic patient against all the everyday risks, but these should be explained to him and to his friends as far as is possible and all precautions should be taken against severe injuries. Careful attention must be paid to the patient's general hygiene.

Moderate exercise is necessary but violent exercise may precipitate an attack. The diet should be ample and contain adequate vitamins. Care must be taken to ensure daily bowel evacuation.

2. During the Fit.—Treatment of a patient in an epileptic attack consists merely in preventing him from injuring himself. The attack is self-limited and no immediate treatment will shorten its course.

3. After the Fit.—Remove all soiled clothing, wash the patient, and put him to bed in a quiet darkened room. Maintain constant observation until he completely recovers consciousness.

5

HYPERKINETIC BEHAVIOUR

This is a condition which results from damage to the cortex of the brain or from destruction of the myelin sheath around nerve-fibres caused by a variety of trauma. It affects boys more often than girls. It occasionally occurs in phenylketonuria and in some cases of drug idiosyncrasies.

It is a distressing condition, leading to complete exhaustion, and it is one that is very demanding of the nurse's tolerance.

The main sign of the condition is excessive motor activity; the child is never at rest and may have only 1 or 2 hours' sleep in 24 hours. He is destructive and vicious towards other patients and the nurses caring for him. His powers of concentration are very poor and he is easily distracted, making play and training extremely difficult. Usually epilepsy accompanies the condition.

Because the source of the attacks originates in the changed cortex of the brain, barbiturates, which are usually the drugs of first choice in epilepsy, would only irritate the condition more. Hydantoinates and primidone therefore become the drugs of choice for the epilepsy, and amphetamine, paraldehyde, and tranquillizers for the excessive motor activity.

Good nursing is essential, and very often the patient needs the services of one nurse to himself as he is unable to form group relationships and is always subject to the dangers of excessive exhaustion and injury, until such time as a drug has been found which will control the excessive motor activity.

CEREBRAL PALSY

Cerebral palsy is characterized by a disorganization of motor control which results from damage to the central nervous system. Cerebral palsy refers to a variety of motor defects with or without athetosis (uncontrolled waving of the limbs) which appear at birth or in early childhood.

There are several causative factors, among them are congenital anomalies of the brain due to defects in the reproductive process, hereditary degenerative diseases of the brain, acquired postnatal abnormalities of the brain, mainly traumatic or infectious in nature, brain injury during birth, and oxygen deprivation before and during birth.

Some children with cerebral palsy have one or more limbs which are rigidly immobilized by muscular contractions. This spastic group is usually classified according to the number of limbs involved :—
1. Monoplegia.
2. Hemiplegia.
3. Triplegia.
4. Quadriplegia.

Others suffer from an excess amount of motor activity such as chorea (rapid, jerky, involuntary movements), and athetosis (slow, worm-like, purposeless movements exaggerated by voluntary action). Other less common muscular disorders include dystonia (muscle tone above or below normal), tremors, and rigidity. A number of patients suffer from ataxia (impairment of postural activity and walking).

The particular type of disruption in motor function depends upon the site and extent of the damage. Spastic symptoms are common when there are lesions in the pyramidal tract of the brain and spinal column causing increasing contraction of the muscles. Athetosis is more likely to result from lesions occurring in the extrapyramidal system, whose effects are normally inhibitory. Some authorities suggest that athetoid symptoms tend to follow anoxia while cerebral hæmorrhage tends to cause spasticity.

Often one of the greatest problems with a cerebrally palsied child who has a severe handicap in motor activity and communication is assessing his intellectual capacity. The special disabilities of the cerebrally palsied child add immeasurably to the severity of whatever intellectual deficiency he may have. Often he has such speech and motor difficulties that he cannot make his wants known and is unable to achieve a sense of independence.

Not all cerebrally palsied children are severely handicapped, many are able to maintain relatively normal lives providing supporting services are available.

THE AUTISTIC CHILD

Most children are uninhibited at first, almost all children cry, kick, scream, bite, and attack their environment directly when it does not give them what they want. Surprisingly early in most children's lives, they learn that a smile, a happy babble, and an occasional change of mind about a demand will gain just as much attention.

The autistic baby fails to reach out to be picked up and remains stiff and unaccommodating in his mother's arms. The pre-school autistic child acts as if other persons were not there and prefers solitude to company. He tends to react as if people were inanimate objects. If his arm is held by an adult for example, he will tear at the offending hand. He can play with some toys for hours, especially manipulative toys, but he is likely to employ them unimaginatively, ignoring the use for which they were intended.

An autistic child's speech is either absent or severely impaired.

The behaviour of the autistic child has much in common with schizophrenia.

The three cardinal symptoms can be classified as follows :—

1. Avoidance of friendly contact.
2. Repetitive preoccupied behaviour.
3. Failure to communicate by speech.

It is usually possible to ascertain the intellectual ability of these children and it is often adequate for learning.

There is no known medical treatment but the emphasis is on 'education' which involves the whole of the child's waking day and providing an individual approach, presenting the child with the opportunity of making use of any sort of material which takes his fancy, and then unobtrusively providing aid and suggestions. I have known a teacher use a child's interest in disposable paper towels to present him with the challenge and opportunity to learn to read and form a friendly relationship with the teacher.

Taking care of such children is one of the most challenging, fascinating, and frequently disheartening tasks in nursing. Its rewards are so few and so infrequent that one can easily become discouraged. The nurse has to give and give and continue to give without wanting any return.

Since these children do not communicate well, the nurse must consider how to communicate with them. The nurse's voice is of great importance and the most important quality in her voice is genuine affection. Children quickly pick up the real warmth and affection which the nurse can show even when she is denying the child something he wants immediately. We are not too aware of how our emotions creep into our voices, even when we pride ourselves on our fine control ; the sigh of impatience we think we have suppressed, the little edginess of irritation, the sharpened pitch when we have been frightened, these show in our voices, and children, especially sick children, seem acutely sensitive to them.

It is not easy to play, or work, with children 8 hours a day, but we can make it easier by not setting up standards that are adult and limiting to children.

There are many things to take into consideration in working with young children. Time is endless to them, it has no great meaning to them. Tomorrow, or later, is something they cannot grasp. Try to plan your day beforehand so that you can help them with such occasions as : now is when we eat breakfast ; then after breakfast we visit the toilet and wash our hands. Try to think as the child does in concrete and small time sequences, with every new experience filled with wonder and curiosity. Accept the child for what he is and recognize his limitations. Prepare him to accept adult standards by making them interesting and fun.

As such, children are entitled to the respect and courtesy one gives to any other human being. The child's small size and lack of social sophistication tend to make adults treat him with amused condescension or as a plaything. Children are neither, they are growing individual persons, and their needs and wants are basically the same as those of adults ; they differ only in their ability to interpret these needs adequately or in a socially acceptable manner.

We must remember many small important things when we work with children, one of which is an actual physical difference in the point of view. Kneel down to a child's height occasionally, the world looks different from there, especially an indoor world of adult-sized furniture and equipment, and kneel down, if you will, to a child's height in thought and action. Children see many things we do not notice from our height, or because we take them for granted.

When dealing with disturbed children, the nurse should ask herself how important and how much routine is necessary. How important is it that the child cleans his teeth, combs his hair, and washes his hands and face? Certainly with disturbed children, it is more important to have a child comfortable and at ease than uneasy and disturbed, and beautifully groomed. Comfortable emotions are so much better than looking nice. The framework of habit-training, eating, and sleeping is important, but the nurse should be flexible within the framework.

One of the most important things we can teach the disturbed child is that we love him; we should say so in words and actions over and over again. The nurse will often need to correct the child but loss of love should never be inferred from her admonishment. If something has annoyed you, do not try to hide it; if you are amused, laugh. But be ready to explain that certain behaviour is not accepted by most people and that you still love him, even if you have to restrict his behaviour. The nurse must be able to pick up an untidy, hostile child and keep him from hurting himself, another child, or the nurse herself, and help him feel that he is not being rejected.

There is no set formula for managing autistic children, but if you genuinely 'like' children you should have no trouble learning what is the correct reaction in a given situation.

There are many problems for the nurse caring for the autistic child, not least is the emotional entanglement she can get into, both with the child and his parents.

The nurse should take time to speak to the parents, show them the ward and the things their child has done, and plans for the child's day. Take time to arrange for the parents to see the doctor or the social worker if they seem to need to do so.

Another danger in this nursing is the great attachment which the nurse may make to the child. It is important that the nurse loves the child, to hold him, pet him, play with him. But the nurse must not let herself become so involved that he becomes her only life.

Despite these risks of involvement, work with the autistic child can be challenging and satisfying. Every day more is being learned about the autistic child and the outlook is more hopeful. It is highly specialized nursing.

The right environment and the right staff can help autistic children to be thawed out and often they are shown to be fundamentally normal children.

SPEECHLESSNESS (MUTISM)

Next to deafness, mental subnormality is probably the most common cause of absence of speech, and if at the age of 2 a child has not developed normal speech, the diagnosis probably rests between mental subnormality and deafness. The more uncommon causes of absence of speech in children are autism and childhood schizophrenia. Temporary mutism may be due to hysteria and it may also be due to the parents' attitude to the child. There are many parents who worry if their child does not speak at an early age and, as a result, continually urge the child to repeat words after them. They become irritable with the child's mistakes, repeatedly correct him, and as a result the child develops a negative attitude towards speech and therefore remains or becomes silent.

Children undergoing prolonged hospitalization often show a delayed onset in speaking, and lack of stimulation is the factor involved. The child who is looked after by his mother and is spoken to by her is helped considerably in his speech development, and at the same time is satisfied emotionally. Where a child has impairment of hearing, sounds are indistinct and, as a result, the child has difficulty in reproducing them and in this way may show faulty articulation.

Another cause of delayed onset of speech is that associated with word deafness or auditory aphasia. As a result of this the child is unable to understand the meaning of the spoken word although he can in fact hear it.

The child goes through the normal babbling period. Later it is noticed that he does not understand simple commands and does not attach the usual meaning to his own utterances, but at the same time can understand and express himself through gestures. If the child finds that the words he uses convey no meaning to others his speech will be restricted to a few sounds.

Insecurity is the sensitive child's worst enemy. This feeling, arising as it may do from emotional shocks in childhood, may be out of all proportion to the circumstances that caused them. What may seem to be a comparatively innocuous incident to an adult may have a severe impact on the mind of a small child initiating his difficulty in learning to speak.

Separation from parents can set up separation-anxiety in a child and inhibit the onset of speech as a reaction.

In trying to help a child to learn to talk, speak slowly and clearly to him, giving him easy words to copy. Choose a time to talk to him when he is most likely to give you his full attention. Avoid being over-eager, even if his slowness is giving concern. Patience in awaiting his clear utterances will be the most rewarding. Try to provoke speech by holding a desired object at arm's length until some vocalization is made. Being given the object afterwards will help him realize the usefulness of speech and encourage further attempts. Once a child has said a word, give him opportunities for repeating it, without confusing him with new words. Repeating a word gives satisfaction to a child and fixes it in his memory.

Aim to build up a feeling of enjoyment and pleasure connected with speech, so that the child wants to communicate with others. Use stories and games to emphasize sounds and words. Never project your own anxiety to the child.

To those who appreciate the need to be able to communicate with others it must be frustrating not to be able to tell others their needs, fears, and anxieties. When speech is absent, the nurse will need to be observant and thorough in her training in order that she may note any behaviour characteristics and relate them to any bodily change of her patient, and she must teach methods of communication through pantomime if speech is impossible. This can be a very interesting and rewarding endeavour.

DEAFNESS

A normal baby is born with the ability to react to sounds. This ability subsequently matures, until by 6 months he should be hearing normally. At first, he responds more readily to noises than to voices though he has some appreciation of the emotional content of his mother's voice. Then as he approaches 6 months a voice begins to mean more to him, especially when it is quiet.

It is not always easy to test deafness, particularly in a mentally subnormal child. An audiometer is a machine used in testing hearing ability. A child who can concentrate and co-operate will be able to respond to an audiometer test and show how loud a sound need be for him to hear it and which pitches he hears better than others. The knowledge gained from this test helps the otologist to plan the best treatment for the child whose hearing is not normal.

With mentally subnormal children one has to rely on careful observations of the child; reactions to sounds, such as the following :—

1. Does a loud noise startle him? A newborn baby will react to a sudden loud noise with the movement of an eyelid or jerk of the body.

2. Does he ever stop crying to listen to a noise that interests him?

3. Does he turn his head or eyes towards the source of sound?

4. Does he respond to speech?

5. Does he fail to look up when spoken to?

6. Does he watch the person's face intently when he listens?

When a child is suspected of having a hearing deficiency he should be referred to an audiometrician.

Hearing-aids are available for children, and although they do not restore hearing they aid partial hearing. Children with sufficient hearing to be familiar with the sounds of speech will benefit immediately from a suitably adjusted hearing-aid. Others with a greater hearing loss may not find it an advantage at all, or will need considerable training in learning to distinguish between, and appreciate the significance of, sounds previously heard.

According to the type of deafness the child will be recommended to use a bone-conduction or an air-conduction earpiece. Only a medical expert can decide upon the most suitable in each case. A bone-conduction ear-piece is worn behind the ear over the mastoid; whereas the air-conduction ear-piece is specially moulded to fit individual ears. The easiest kind of aid for a mentally subnormal child to wear is the transistor type which is neat and small with batteries enclosed.

When a child has been issued with a hearing-aid the nurse's attitude to its use is most important; if she considers it to be a nuisance, so will the child; if she welcomes it and compliments him on his own little radio he will probably be pleased to wear it.

Children who do not hear properly can be very awkward. They are frequently tense and uncoordinated in their movements. They are frustrated by their inability to hear what others say and to express their own thoughts articulately. They sometimes become withdrawn, refusing to make friends with other children, and suppressing their desires to listen, understand, and communicate. Frustrations are often more keenly felt by children with partial hearing than by the severely deaf. Tempers are a common occurrence but are at least an expression of communication and means of working off frustrated feelings. Toys that allow play to be aggressive such as banging toys, etc., are beneficial.

BLINDNESS

Blindness is a relatively common affliction amongst the mentally subnormal population; its causative factor usually being that which has caused the mental subnormality. It is not unusual for the blind child to be also deaf. Impaired vision is also common and often in the past it was unnoticed.

Today, with so much emphasis being placed on rehabilitation it is difficult for these serious afflictions not to be diagnosed and treatment given where appropriate. Absence of sight should not of its own limit the learning capacity of the child; with patient training techniques it is possible for this child to develop a satisfying life, and provided the contents of his environment do not change too frequently, his mobility and independence will develop to satisfying degrees.

The nurse should, as far as possible, avoid all reference to the patient's disability and instead endeavour to encourage the development of independence. Once he has been assisted around his new home and been introduced to the other patients, he should be allowed to make his own friends and to find his own way around.

The child's education should not be limited because of his lack of sight, but like all other of his physical requirements should be brought to maximum maturity.

Blindness evokes a great deal of public sympathy. The nurse must at all costs avoid becoming too emotionally involved, otherwise her judgement will become clouded and her work and effort detrimentally affected. Never let the patient feel that you have this excess of sympathy for him, otherwise he will become increasingly demanding and dependent, which will in turn prolong his rehabilitation.

PHYSICAL HANDICAPS

Patients who, two decades ago, were dying in early life are now living longer. This means that those with severe physical disabilities present a nursing-care problem for many more years. In the past emphasis was placed on survival rather than on training. Now we must recognize the patient's right to learn self-care habits and to develop his potential for independence by functional training and through being given opportunities to develop skills in self-care such as in feeding, habit training, and locomotion. All these are of value as every skill learned leads to less care being needed, to more independence, and to less behaviour problems such as noisy outbursts, masturbation, and sucking parts of the body. Success in any one of the skills gives the patient a great boost to his morale and motivates him for more learning.

Self-feeding.—Experimentation with feeding utensils and modifications of stock issue may be necessary to achieve results. Very often a scientifically minded nurse is able to reduce the difficulties to a minimum.

Self-feeding by these patients will be messy and more prolonged than when the nurse feeds the patient. However, she should not let this influence her training. Patience and encouragement will be needed from time to time.

It will be found that the health of these patients will improve and easier management will be facilitated if the tendency towards excess weight is avoided.   Careful supervision of their diet will need to be constant.

Habit Training.—Every effort should be made to encourage use of the normal toilets in the manner of the ambulant patients.   In order to eliminate some of the difficulties it may be necessary to have some minor alterations made to existing toilets.   For instance, toilets need to be spacious to allow movement of invalid chairs and the assistance of one or two nurses.   Toilet pans need to be of a convenient height with arm-rests to support the transfer of the patient from his chair to the pan and vice versa.   The flushing system should be so placed that the patient can reach it without effort.   Patients should not be left sitting on the lavatory pan too long at any one time.   The patient will need a great deal of encouragement and reassurance if constipation is to be avoided.   The nurse must therefore make every effort to introduce regular habit training as soon as possible.

Locomotion.—To be able to move about allows the patient to explore and make use of his environment.   It is possible, through the agency of the Ministry of Social Security, for invalid wheel chairs to be supplied to individual patients on a medical prescription.   Other locomotion aids made available are : special light-weight walking sticks which are adjustable in height, walking aids, and surgical boots.   There are occasions when surgical boots serve no real purpose ; all that is required is a covering for the feet to keep out the weather.

PHYSIOTHERAPY

Many mentally subnormal patients have in the past been nursed as helpless bed patients, thus incapacitating them still further physically, which in turn will prevent any future effort of rehabilitation.

Contractures of the upper and lower limbs and spine were previously considered to be concomitant with many of the individual clinical types and hemiplegias.   With our improved knowledge we now know that this is not so and that many of the physical deformities can be prevented, providing early measures are taken, such as correct body mechanics, proper positioning of the patient in bed, early attempts at ambulation, and corrective and preventive exercises.

The body is made of movable joints that are found in the spine, the shoulders, the elbows, the wrists and fingers, the hips, the knees, the ankles, and the toes. Every activity of the daily life is dependent upon the ability of the joints to move freely, and any limitation of range of movement in the joints interferes with normal function of the parts.

In order to assist with the prevention of deformity it is important that the nurse knows the normal range of motion in the joints of the shoulders, elbows, wrists, fingers, hips, knees, ankles, toes, and spinal column.

There are 9 different kinds of movements to the various movable joints of the body. These movements are flexion, extension, hyperextension, abduction, adduction, internal rotation, external rotation, pronation, and supination. The joints of the shoulders and hips use the first 7 of these movements. The movements of the elbow joints are flexion, extension, pronation, and supination. The knee joints have 2 movements—flexion and extension. The wrists have 4 : flexion, extension, pronation, and supination ; the ankles have 4 : flexion, extension, internal rotation, and external rotation. There are 2 movements in the joints of the toes—flexion and extension ; in the fingers there are 4 : flexion, extension, abduction, and adduction. The spinal column also contains movable joints ; those of the cervical and lumbar spine are capable of 3 movements—flexion, extension, and rotation.

A contracture is a permanent shortening of muscle-fibres. When a muscle becomes shortened or contracted there may be changes and distortion in bone structure ; thus a deformity is produced.

What then can nurses do to prevent contracture deformities? The nurse must acquire a thorough understanding of posture techniques, and she must develop the ability to apply the principles of good body alinement and correct positioning of the patient in bed or chair. She must know when and how to use mechanical aids (sandbags, etc.) to secure correct positioning of the patient in bed under the direction of the doctor.

The nurse must be an enthusiastic advocate of corrective exercising and early ambulation.

In general, corrective exercising is primarily a function of the physiotherapists who are trained in this science. Where physiotherapists are available, a programme of exercises should be outlined under the direction of a doctor and initiated by the physiotherapist. The nurse, however, properly supervised by the physiotherapist, may perform many of the activities thus outlined. But, in the absence of qualified personnel, and under medical direction, the nurse may perform and may teach the patient to perform many of the simpler exercises that will aid in the prevention of physical deformities. Therefore it is essential that nurses understand some of the basic principles of physiotherapy.

Exercises may be active or passive. Active exercises are performed by the wilful action of the patient. Passive exercises are exercises performed by an operator or mechanical agent without the assistance or resistance of the patient. Exercises performed by means of the hands of the physiotherapist are passive exercises because they involve movement of muscles without the assistance of the patient.

Active and passive exercises have been divided into three groups according to their function :—

1. Exercises that are used to maintain general muscle tone in unaffected parts of the body.

2. Exercises that are used to strengthen normal muscles.

3. Exercises that are used to strengthen and re-educate diseased or injured muscles.

The principles of corrective, remedial, or preventive exercises should be incorporated into nursing care, because they help to maintain good muscle tone and strengthen normal muscles that may atrophy from disuse. They play an integral part in rendering physically handicapped patients less handicapped and in preventing irreversible contractures.

WHEEL CHAIRS

When it is indicated that a handicapped person in the home or in the hospital will need to use a wheel chair part or all of the time, a type of chair should be provided that is adapted to the patient's height, weight, physical disability, doorway width, passageways, and hallways. A collapsible chair that can be folded for automobile transportation and for storage where space is limited is desirable.

A wheel chair gives the handicapped person an opportunity for active normal living, for enjoyment of outside interests, and for personal freedom and independence.

CHAPTER V

THE ADMISSION OF A PATIENT

WHEN admitting a patient to hospital the nurse must consider both his psychological and physical needs. She should also have a knowledge of his family background, which is very important.

ATTITUDE ON ADMISSION

Psychological Needs.—During his development a child has certain basic needs such as adequate nourishment, clothing, and shelter. Equally vital is his need for affection and a feeling of security within the family group. The love of his mother is the child's most important requirement, and in the absence of a mother, a mother-substitute is necessary to take her place.

When a mentally subnormal person is sent to hospital, he is usually being separated from his mother for the first time in his life. He will receive all the specialized care available, but unless the nurse does her best in every way to prove a substitute for the mother the child will fret and show emotional upsets, as would a normal child. He may fret openly and be inconsolable in his tears, or inwardly and become quiet, withdrawn, and morose. Consider how a subnormal child must feel when he loses contact with maternal warmth and security. His security has been undermined, he is struggling to overcome a wave of depressing grief, and he is confused and bewildered in his loyalty to his mother, who, it would seem, has committed him to a strange environment amidst a host of strangers.

No normal child likes to feel that he is loved only on a selective basis. Almost unconsciously he is driven to test by provocative behaviour the affection offered to him. He is

PLATE II

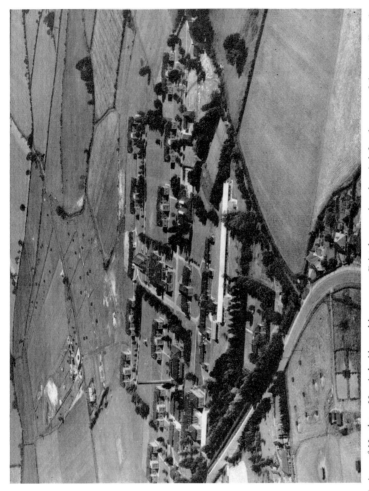

Aerial view of Hortham Hospital, Almondsbury, near Bristol, a modern hospital for the care of the mentally subnormal.

(By courtesy of Aero Pictorial Ltd., London.)

PLATE III

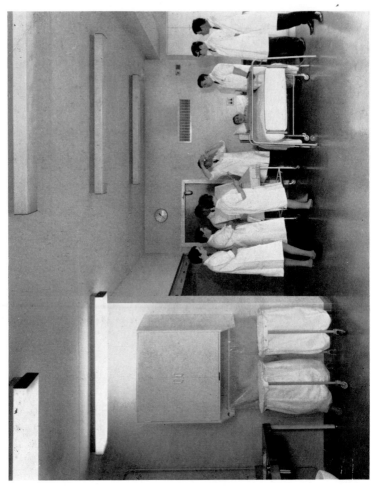

'School of Nursing', Lynebank Hospital, Dunfermline   Class in progress.

(By courtesy of the Stratheden and Associated Hospital Board of Management.)

finding out for himself if he will be loved while he remains co-operative and well behaved, and rejected when naughty and disobedient. By deliberately provoking adults he is judging the reactions of those who promise affection and security. If he is still accepted when he is badly behaved, he feels he can safely put his trust in those who are caring for him. If they satisfy the patient's psychological needs he will develop a state of mind which will enable him to accept the problems and disappointments he receives in his daily life. It is important that he is accepted by his group, as this will be an important stabilizing influence.

When a nurse admits a new patient to her ward the formalities should be kept to a minimum. The importance of first impressions must not be overlooked. The unconscientious nurse will merely fill in the form of particulars, transport the patient to his ward and bed, and casually dismiss the parents. The nurse *should*, however, be sympathetic and recognize the parents' problems, which will in all probability be of an emotional nature. It must be remembered that the mother is bringing her own flesh and blood into a hospital which cares for the mentally subnormal child. She realizes that there may be no cure available and that as a result her child may have to spend the rest of his life in such a place.

Most of the parents, because they have not been forewarned, have been unable to act decisively ; because of their lack of knowledge of mental subnormality they do not appreciate the true nature of their problem.

Following the birth of a subnormal child the parents may spend many anxious years searching for help and true guidance. Even after having her child admitted to hospital, the mother still requires reassuring. The nurse can do much to give the parent peace of mind and in return for this she may ask for her full co-operation. Nurses have a wonderful opportunity to be of service to these people in their hour of need. Parent and patient should be received with expectancy and a friendly welcome. One method of approach to the patient and relatives is first of all for the nurse to take time to introduce herself to them properly, never appearing to hurry, and to address them by name if their names are known to her. The

6

first meeting can have a lasting effect and it does help the patient to feel that he is not a stranger. Opportunity for parents and patient to look round the patient's new home together should be arranged and the mother should be given an insight into the care and training her child will receive. Not until a firm, friendly foundation has been prepared between the nurse and parent should any conditions or instructions be given. Once a mother's confidence is gained it will be easy for her to accede to the hospital's wishes. Visiting days and hours of visiting, times of buses and the number of the bus, the telephone number of the hospital, suggestions about food parcels and clothing, and any other information parents may need should be given clearly.

It is the rule in some hospitals for parents to visit the hospital before their child is admitted. There is much to be commended in this system, as it tends to break down the parents' fears of the unknown before their child is admitted.

Physical Needs.—Early in the period of welcoming the new patient, the nurse must ascertain whether he has had a recent meal. If not, arrangements must be made to provide him with an appetizing meal as soon as possible. Quite often all that is required is a friendly welcome, attention to small needs, and possibly a picture-book to interest him for the moment.

Once the patient has settled down and gained confidence in his surroundings he can be bathed in the manner Sister considers most suitable. It is usually necessary to help him in this, and vital relationships can be strengthened if the nurse shows tact and thoughtfulness during the carrying out of the procedure. Any obvious physical abnormality can easily be noted while the patient is being bathed, and should be reported to the Ward Sister as soon as he has been made comfortable in bed.

Discretion should be used as to whether the patient's hair is fine tooth-combed or not. If such a duty has to be carried out, a little tactful explanation will be necessary in the case of patients who are likely to feel embarrassment over it; it will in most cases prevent surprised indignation.

The bed to which the patient is taken after his bath should be clean, warmed, and invitingly turned down. These simple but important finishing touches will help him to gain confidence in his surroundings and in the nursing staff responsible for his care. When the patient expresses a desire to visit the toilet, it is usual to collect a specimen of urine for a routine test.

OBSERVATION OF CHARACTERISTICS

During the days immediately after admission it will be important to note the following characteristics and report on them as necessary :—

1. Health Habits.—

Breathing.—The correct way to breathe is through the nose, not the mouth. Patients suffering from a deflected septum, enlarged adenoids, or catarrh will breathe through the mouth because of the difficulty experienced with nose breathing.

Sleep.—A record of the patient's sleep should include observations on its duration and character. Is it restful or fitful? Is there difficulty in getting off to sleep? Do dreams and nightmares disturb the sleep? Does the patient appear to be rested on waking in the morning?

Toilet Habits.—Regularity of bowel action, frequency of micturition, and whether these functions are carried out with ease or if they cause distress should be noted. Are the toilet habits clean or do they require correction ?

Eating Habits.—Some patients bolt their food without properly chewing it, others may be more particular and be slow and methodical in their eating. The nurse must make sure that every patient has adequate time allowed for eating his food. It may be necessary to seat all those who are slow eaters together to make it easier for the nurse to pay attention to them. A report should be submitted on the quantity of food a new patient eats, and whether he shows a lack of interest in it. He will show his mechanical and dextrous ability in his handling of cutlery at meal times.

Personal Cleanliness.—Most patients take a pride in their appearance if given encouragement. Where this encouragement has been missing in their previous environment, it may be found that they respond with a slovenly, untidy appearance.

From these early observations the nurse is made aware of the extent of her task in the health education of her patients.

2. Physical Symptoms.—

Bruises.—These must be noticed early and reported immediately.

Complexion.—Notice whether the face is flushed, pale, or cyanosed.

Cough.—Any cough is significant and must be reported.

Discharges.—Report any discharge from any orifice.

Excitement and Overactiveness.—A report on these may direct attention towards a possible superimposed mental state.

Excreta.—Observations on the excretion of fæces and urine and on expectoration should include the amount, colour, and smell ; any incontinence should be reported also.

Inflammation.—The presence of redness and swelling of a part should be reported upon immediately so that treatment can be instituted without delay.

Menstruation.—Irregularity or absence of the menstrual periods amongst female mentally subnormal patients is common. The duration, amount, character, odour, and any accompanying discomfort or pain should be reported.

Temperature.—Slight variations occur according to the time of day or the amount of exercise taken, the normal range being between 97° F. and 99° F. The temperature of a mentally subnormal patient should be taken in the axilla, care being taken that the axilla is dry and that the bulb of the thermometer is between folds of skin and not clothing.

Pulse.—Wherever an artery is near the surface of the body and crosses over a bone, the wave of blood can be felt and is called a pulse. The nurse should note its frequency, regularity, and fullness, and the condition of the artery.

Weight.—A very important record, which through any abnormal variation in weight will indicate the state of the patient's health.

3. Speech.—Abnormalities of speech are common among mentally subnormal patients, and may be due to defective hearing or functional ability.

Defective Hearing.—A patient who from birth has been unable to hear will also be unable to speak owing to lack of experience of the spoken word. Deafness occurring before the age of 7 years will have the same results. The vocabulary acquired at that age is so small as to be useless, and is easily forgotten unless special teaching is instituted early.

Defective Functional Ability.—Anatomical defects, such as cleft palate, hare lip, and muscular and nervous conditions will cause any of the following disabilities :—

a. Aphonia : The patient is unable to speak louder than a whisper in spite of his efforts to strengthen his voice.

b. Stammering : A muscular spasm prevents and interrupts speech.

c. Stuttering : Repetition of the sounds of individual vowels and consonants.

d. General defects : These can take the form of very slow or rapid speech, with the omission of syllables, or slurring, stumbling over, or separation of them.

e. Defective development of the speech centre : The ability to speak largely depends upon the development of the brain. If, as in more severely subnormal patients, it fails to develop beyond that of a baby, attempts at speech will be no more than noise-making, but with higher degrees of mental development there will be an accompanying higher level of speech ability. The following defects may occur :—

Lalling : This is the term used to describe an infantile, babbling form of speech.

Idioglossia : In this condition the patient is trying to evade difficulties by inventing his own speech.

Agrammatism : The patient ignores the grammatical structure of the language.

Lisping : The substitution of ' th ' sounds for ' s ', ' sh ', and ' z '.

Echolalia : The question is repeated before the answer is given.

Coprolalia : Pouring out a stream of obscene expressions.

Verbigeration : Endless repetition of a word or phrase which does not appear to have any meaning.

4. Gait.—In studying the gait the points to be noted, if the patient can walk, are : Does he walk straight ? Can he follow a straight line ? Does he tend to fall ? If so, in what direction ?

The chief types of abnormal gait are :—

a. Spastic.—The patient has difficulty in bending his knees and drags his feet along, the toes scraping the ground at each step. This condition may affect one or both legs, and is seen in lesions of the pyramidal tracts and hemiplegia.

b. Stamping or Ataxia.—The patient raises his feet abnormally high, then jerks them forward, bringing them to the ground with a stamp, heel first. If he watches the ground with his eyes he will be fairly steady, but if he closes his eyes he will lose his balance.

c. Drunken or Reeling.—These patients walk with their feet planted widely apart 'on a broad base'. This gait is similar to the one adopted by a person under the influence of alcohol or narcotic drugs.

d. Festinant or Tripping.—The patient is bent forwards and advances with rapid, short, shuffling steps as if he were trying to catch the centre of gravity. He does not swing his arms. Sometimes he will start walking backwards and is unable to stop himself. This is known as retropulsion, and is associated with encephalitis lethargica.

e. Waddling or Oscillating.—This resembles the walk of a duck, the body being tilted backwards. It is met with in lordosis of the lumbar spine and congenital dislocation of the hip.

5. Muscular Co-ordination.—By muscular co-ordination is meant the harmonious working of separate muscles or groups of muscles in order to carry out a definite function. If this co-operation is absent or imperfect the carrying out of the function becomes difficult and without rhythm, or it becomes impossible.

Curvatures of the Spine.—The curvature may be in an anterior, posterior, or lateral direction. An abnormal forward curve in the lumbar spine is called lordosis. A posterior curvature of the spine is known as kyphosis or ' hunchback '. An abnormal lateral deviation of the spine is called scoliosis.

6. Interests.—Once a knowledge of a patient's interests is gained, the gateway to rehabilitation is open. Conversation will be the main channel through which potential interests will be discovered. In thinking of the patient as a person, his home, his life, his experiences, and the things he likes or enjoys are important, and they will help in understanding him.

When planning conversation it is important to appreciate when it is out of place and what subjects are dangerous. Intelligent silence and attentive listening will often produce equally satisfying results.

7. Activity.—Does the patient move quickly and rhythmically or are his movements slow and lethargic ? Is he alert or does he sit in a corner with apparent lack of interest ? Often it seems impossible to arouse interest in a patient who is antagonistic towards all the nurse's efforts. The preliminary step is to make activity necessary. Regardless of the patient's behaviour, the nurse should keep working towards objectives that are in the patient's reach.

8. Sociability.—The nurse's report on her patient should contain a record of his attitude towards other patients and staff. For instance, does he take an interest in his surroundings ? Does he associate with other patients and join in their games, or does he remain apart ? Does he accept authority, or is he aggressive towards anyone representing it ?

CHAPTER VI

METHODS OF EXAMINATION AND INVESTIGATION OF THE MENTALLY SUBNORMAL

THE examination of a mentally subnormal person differs from other types of examination, and it should be carried out in two parts whenever possible : (1) Without supervision ; (2) With relatives present.

During the examination it should be discovered what capacity the patient has for caring for himself without supervision and what degrees of self-care he can achieve with supervision.

METHOD OF EXAMINATION

1. **History.**—There may be an absence of reliable subjective information from the patient himself, depending upon the degree of subnormality. The examiner therefore has to depend upon other means to provide him with important facts. The doctor himself is ultimately responsible for getting the history but he usually delegates the responsibility to the social worker who is specially trained in this capacity. The use of a social worker to take the social history has many advantages. It relieves the doctor of the necessity to devote time to fact-finding and leaves him time to use more profitably in examining the patient. It enables the social worker to visit the home and helps her to enter into a relationship with the family. Taking a social history is an art and requires great skill and patience. The whole process is fraught with difficulties. The relatives may not have appreciated sufficiently the significance of developmental landmarks to have noted them, or they may have forgotten them. In families where there are three or four children important facts may be ascribed to one or other

of the children. Some parents in their anxiety and desire to make their offspring appear brighter than he actually is will unknowingly distort the facts, while others may exaggerate their difficulties and distort them in other ways.

a. Personal History.—This should be a very comprehensive report and no detail about the patient should be dismissed without consideration as being unimportant. It should contain information about :—

i. *Birth of the patient* : Place of birth in the family, age of parents, mother's state during pregnancy, whether she had a normal delivery or whether it was accompanied by some abnormality, the appearance of the child at birth, whether it breathed normally or whether there was some delay.

ii. *Progress through childhood* : A record outlining the milestones of his progress should be made, for instance : feeding, the age at which he smiled, raised his head, sat up, crawled, and walked alone ; the age at which he was weaned, when he talked, and when he became toilet trained ; behaviour and personality as a toddler and pre-school behaviour.

iii. *School and nursery reports* : These reports are considered and should include the age of entry and the age of leaving. The child's degree of competence in handling subjects taught, and any truancy, maladjustment, or unsociability recorded during his school-going career.

iv. *Self-care* : It is important to report on the child's habits as fully as possible. The nature of these will give an indication of his self-care ability.

v. *Separation* : There may have been factors necessitating the separation of the child from his mother or of the mother's own inability to tolerate physical contact. In such cases the reason and the duration should be investigated.

vi. *Employability* : The nature of his employment and the reasons why changes have taken place if they have happened.

vii. *Previous health* : What physical illnesses and accidents has he had and at what age did they occur? It is important that the following be reported upon in detail : Meningitis, concussion, fainting attacks, chorea, venereal disease, epilepsy, and any of the virus infections.

viii. *Circumstances leading to admission* : Whether due to change in family circumstances or if due to the patient's misbehaviour and the nature of this.

b. Family History.—Relationship and any great disparity in ages of parents should be noted. Inquiry into the temperament, and for signs of mental instability in either parent, should be made. Are there any cases in the family of eccentricity, insanity, suicide, criminality, mental subnormality, alcoholism, fits, or paralysis ? Has either parent ever contracted syphilis ?

2. Information.—Information is largely acquired through the combined efforts of the doctor, the nurse, and social worker.

A careful routine physical examination is of great importance, and investigation of all systems should be directed towards ascertaining the existence of malnutrition, disease, deformity, or special-sense defect which might be responsible for mental subnormality, and to detect the presence of developmental anomalies and stigmata.

a. The Skin.—The state of the skin will suggest the patient's ability to provide his own self-care or that of others to provide it for him ; information relating to the standard of his general nutrition, if his diet is adequate, or if too much of one class of food is being given and too little of others.

b. Hearing.—If the patient is being examined for deafness, it is important that he is also examined for high-frequency deafness. This could quite easily be the cause of his lack of mental development.

c. Sight.—Though the patient can see, it may be that he can only see things in detail when they are at a certain distance away from him, and he may as a result miss quite a lot of intellectual information without anyone being aware of it.

d. Central Nervous System.—A full and thorough examination of this system is important as it may have an underlying degenerative disease which may not have affected the more recent generations of the family, but is nevertheless present in the family tree.

Other facts concerning the patient's reactions, degree of subnormality, and feeling tone are equally important and need observing so that an accurate assessment can be made.

The points to be noted on interview with the patient are :—

i. How well developed is his speech, whether he can use words in their right context, and whether his vocabulary is extensive or limited.

ii. Is the patient relaxed and at ease during the interview, or does he appear to be insecure and strained ?

iii. What account can he give of himself ?   For instance, can he say when he had his last meal, and what he had for it ? Which school did he go to, what subjects did he do, and with what success ?   What information can he give of his friends and his work ?   All these questions will have to be prepared and presented according to the patient's age and obvious ability.

iv. Is the patient orientated as to time and place?   Does he understand what day, and the time of the day it is, and does he appreciate where he is ?

v. Routine questions such as the patient's name, age, address, etc., are asked.

vi. General information questions are asked to see if the patient is as well informed as a normal child of his age should be, or to gauge the degree of subnormality present.   Questions will include those of everyday usage, such as money sense— if he goes into a shop to buy an article costing 5 new pence with a 10 n.p. piece, how much change will he have ?   In what day and in which year is he living ?   His sense of numbers will also be tested by asking him to multiply 2×2 and subtract 2 from 4.

vii. The patient's 'feeling tone' will be investigated by observing his mood.   Is it in keeping with his circumstances? Is he anxious, depressed, or elated?   Is he suffering from a psychosis masquerading as mental subnormality ?   Has the patient the ability to form a relationship with the examiner, or does he remain flat and uninterested ?

viii. The examiner will get the patient to explain any statements made about him by others, especially with regard to impulsive actions, eccentricities of conduct, moral lapses, etc. An attempt will be made to trace out each symptom to its origin.

3. Objective Information.—This information is given by any or all of the following people who have direct and close contact with the patient : the parents of the patient ; the Sister in charge of the patient's ward ; and the occupational therapist. The information so submitted deals with the same aspects of the patient's abilities, progress, or regression. The points dealt with below are continually being observed, assessed, and reported upon.

a. Capacity for Self-care.—
i. *Feeding* : Can the patient feed himself ? If so, what degree of efficiency can he attain ? Lack of manipulative power, such as being unable to raise the spoon to his mouth, may indicate spasticity and athetosis.

ii. *Dressing* : The degree of skill he achieves in dressing and undressing himself with or without assistance, and the manipulative power of his hands in fastening his buttons, shoe-laces, etc.

b. Physical Ability.—Reports on the power of the patient's muscular co-ordinations are necessary. If the patient can walk, does he do so with a normal gait ? Can he run and climb ?

c. Intellectual Ability.—Speech is important and it can vary in degree of efficiency amongst the mentally subnormal. All aspects of the patient's ability to use this special sense should be reported upon. Does he speak distinctly, and is his speech normal ? How great is his vocabulary ? Are short phrases used in an attempt to overcome the difficulties of speech ? The ability to read and write, though not essential for self-care, is nevertheless important, and the degree of competency in reading, writing, and spelling should be investigated.

d. Working Ability.—What degree of working efficiency has the patient achieved ? What kind of work does he like doing best ? What skill has he acquired in handling tools associated with his work ?

e. Relationships.—Notes on the patient's relationships with other patients. What is his attitude towards his social life ? Is he solitary or sociable ? Interested or uninterested in other people ? Has he an equable temperament or does he suffer from temper tantrums ? Is he simple, docile, and tractable ?

f. Social Activities.—Does the patient enjoy taking part in social activities? If so, what type? Active or passive? Or does he prefer to watch other people taking part in them?

g. General Work Record.—This report will only be necessary for those patients working away from the hospital and should include the patient's capacity for accepting reasonable authority and whether he is amenable to or hostile towards authority.

4. Special Investigations.—These are carried out for diagnostic purposes and include : (1) Intelligence and personality tests ; (2) School reports ; (3) Electro-encephalography ; (4) Blood analysis ; (5) Urine analysis, including chromatography ; (6) Buccal smears ; (7) Chromosomal investigation ; (8) Hormonal investigation ; (9) Intelligence tests.

Ward reports are prepared on each patient twice a year, by the Sister in charge of the ward. They will include all the special points outlined earlier in this chapter, or any others that affect the patient.

The bi-annual reports keep the Responsible Medical Officers informed of the patient's state, and ensure that no patient is overlooked when he is due for reclassification.

EARLY SIGNS OF MENTAL SUBNORMALITY

All the procedures described in this chapter have the common aim of securing information so that the diagnosis can be soundly based. Though it is important to make a diagnosis of mental subnormality as early in life as possible, it is only possible to do this in the early months of life in the cases where there are gross deformities and in certain metabolic disorders. It is estimated that, of the cases recognizable at birth, between 70 and 80 per cent are either born dead or die within the first few days, and those that survive are usually severely subnormal. However, it is highly important that an early diagnosis is made in such cases as the metabolic disorders, phenylketonuria, galactosæmia, etc., and in the case of cretinism. It is possible to make an early diagnosis in these cases, and prompt treatment has the possibility of success. Mild cases of mental subnormality tend to go unnoticed until the child begins to show failure in school, and some even escape notice until they are at work, when their social incapacity becomes apparent due to their rapid changeover of jobs and frequent involvement with the police. Greater efforts are being made to reduce the number of the mentally subnormal people who are escaping notice.

THE GENERAL CHARACTERISTICS OF THE MENTALLY SUBNORMAL

Subnormal children usually show an all-round retardation of growth patterns. Thus, the babies are small at birth, many are premature, and a number show bodily developmental anomalies. Infant feeding may be hard to establish, and all the motor and other developmental landmarks are late in being passed. In many ways subnormal children will appear to be much younger than their chronological age suggests, but this can be misleading, because there are important qualitative differences too between the retarded and the normal. For example, an eager interest in the future is not common among the subnormal. The inferiority of mind and body will usually be reflected in the individual's appearance. Physique will tend to be poor and size small, or, if large, subnormals will usually be clumsy and dysplastic in build. The presence of skeletal deformities and other defects will add to other peculiarities of appearance. However, much of the dreary appearance of subnormal people will be due to inadequate care. Though they are rarely considered good-looking, well-proportioned, athletic, or graceful in their movements, in many cases their inferiority will not strike the eye if care has been taken with their appearance.

The most outstanding general characteristics of the mental state of subnormal people are their pronounced weakness of instinctual impulse which is revealed in their slow patterns of mental development and acquisition of new skills, in their lack of interest in the environment, and particularly in their lack of persistence in the face of difficulties.

Many exhibit a degree of excitability and a tendency to violence which are not usually encountered among normal children.

All new development and learning is difficult for them and they have little persistence. They are, therefore, repeatedly exposed to situations which they cannot control and which will cause them to regress in their level of behaviour. In the case of the more severely subnormal, the individual will be correspondingly more restricted. The mental level may be less than that of a mental age of 2 years. There is an important difference between the adult with the mental age of 2 and the average 2-year-old child, in that the former has nothing of the capacity of the latter for learning. Severely subnormal individuals are usually incurious, self-satisfied, unaware of what they are missing. They do best in an environment which has been structured for them, in which they have been equipped by patient training to meet recurring daily situations with confidence, and in which help is always forthcoming for the unforeseen incident. Severely subnormal people need to have a code to live by, and to be governed by regulations in all activities of life.

When all the evidence of the physical, clinical, and psychological examinations is complete a consistent pattern of mental subnormality will become evident. The subnormality may not be to the same degree in all functional abilities, because quantity of social experience and the wisdom with which the child has been handled in the family will make enormous differences, particularly to social development and the use of language.

Whatever the variations, the overall state must be one of retardation for the diagnosis of mental subnormality to be valid.

DIAGNOSIS AND PROGNOSIS

Though the family and personal history and the physical condition of the patient give valuable information to the investigator, it is upon his mental state, the degree of development of his mind, and his social capacity that a final diagnosis is made.

DIAGNOSIS

The diagnosis of the various grades of mental subnormality is as follows :—

Severe Subnormality.—The degree of mental retardation of these patients varies from being so far retarded and behind normal standards that they are in need of care and protection against common physical dangers such as falling downstairs or into the fire; they may need assistance to walk and may have no power of speech. At meal times they will either feed themselves with great difficulty, spilling the food around and on themselves, or they will need to be fed. They will possess little or no self-care ability—the nurse will have to wash and dress them and take them to the toilet. These patients will have no understanding of what is going on around them and will show only a limited interest. Music will attract their attention and they will respond to affection from the nurse. Often these patients have other congenital defects.

At the top level of severe subnormality, the patient is unable to manage himself or his affairs. He needs supervision during dressing and washing even though he can perform these duties himself. He shows no initiative in self-care, the lead has always to come from the nurse. At meal times, providing the food is cut up into convenient sizes, he can feed himself with a spoon, but he has no manipulative skill for using a knife and fork.

His toilet habits may be dirty and he may be incontinent, but it is possible through habit training to teach him to be clean and dry. Simple routine tasks which do not require initiative are within his capabilities, provided he is given constant supervision, and that he is not expected to work out any problems which may arise. These patients can speak but will only use short simple phrases. They will memorize words which are used frequently in their hearing and will use them without understanding their meaning. Reading and writing are beyond their capabilities, coins are recognized without appreciation of their true value.

Knowledge of everyday information is completely missing. To the unscrupulous person, this patient is easy prey without his being aware of it.

Subnormality.—This grade of patient varies from the one who has little knowledge of small coinage. He can read a few words and may be able to write one or two words including his name. He can tell the time, his age, and date of birthday, and with a struggle he may know his home

PLATE IV

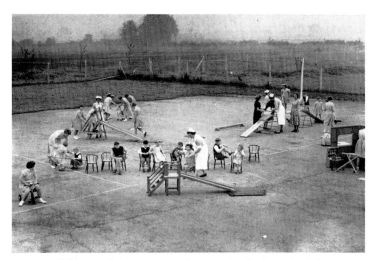

Children at play in a spacious playground at Hortham Hospital.
(By courtesy of the ' Bristol Evening Post '.)

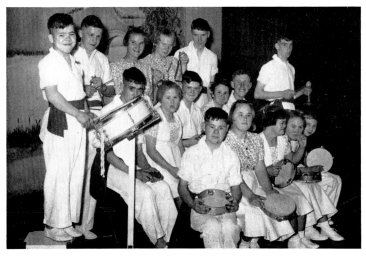

Patients' percussion band at Hortham Hospital.
(By courtesy of the ' Bristol Evening Post '.)

PLATE V

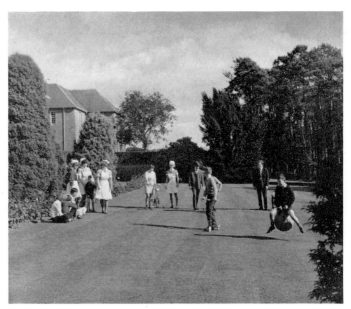

Children at play.

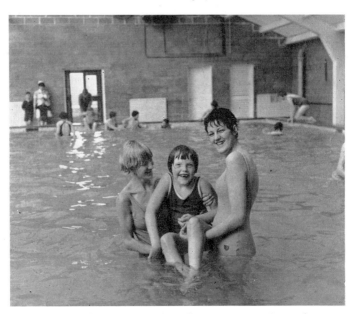

Enjoying the therapeutic values of a spacious swimming pool.
(*Plates V–IX are by courtesy of the Board of Management, Strathmarine Hospital, Dundee.*)

address, but will have no idea of the distance of his home from the hospital. The mildly subnormal patient merges into the normal population, though usually due to his feeling of inferiority he has difficulty in making friends.

The following diagnostic aids will be of assistance :—

Lack of capacity for insight ; the patient is unable to foresee the consequences of some of his actions. He lacks the capacity for abstract thought, for unless he can have something he can see and feel, it will have little meaning for him.

Inability to plan. If, for instance, the patient was given a pint of water which had to last him all day, at the first indication of thirst he would drink the whole of the pint without any thought of his needs for the remainder of the day.

The patient's mind is easily taken off things that matter, and without supervision he will leave a trail of unfinished work, because of poor work habits. He has a serious lack of general knowledge and may also be subjected to emotional instability.

A combination of the above characteristics will give a true concept of the degree of subnormality. The patient can read fairly well from simple books and papers, but he will have difficulty in relating what he has read. He has ability to work with simple sums of money, but lacks planning power. For instance, he may see something which attracts him and he will buy it irrespective of its cost, completely overlooking the fact that he has to pay for other things, such as groceries and rent.

He is unable to adapt himself to new circumstances and will therefore take what, to us, is the easy way out, but to him is the only way out. The patient can carry out all self-care skill with very little supervision and can, to a certain extent, choose his own clothes. He is unable to use his initiative, and if his responsibilities increase he will break down rapidly.

It has been found that very few patients are so subnormal as to be unable to gain some benefit from their training, even though it may only be in the habits of cleanliness and the curtailing of destructive and aggressive behaviour. It has also been realized that there is no cure available which

7

renders the mentally subnormal person able to compete on an equal footing with the normal population.

As with normal children, the mentally subnormal patient is more able to develop his potentialities if training is begun early in life, and if proper training is not given in the early years, maximum development cannot be expected. Mental development in the mentally subnormal patient comes to an end earlier than in a normal person. The subnormal patient should, after a period of training in hospital, be able to lead a happy life in the community with moderate supervision. His chance of acquiring a job and holding it down is poor. A few could manage in a sheltered industry, but in a competitive market would be unable to hold their own. Simple routine tasks in the home are in most cases the best that can be hoped for. The prognosis for the mildly subnormal patient depends upon the type of person who is going to look after him, the degree of responsibility he is going to have, his degree of emotional stability, his social adjustment, and his attitude to reasonable discipline.

Psychopathic Disorder.—The psychopathically disordered person usually shows a complete disregard for the rules, regulations, and demands of society. His social and personal relationships are also disordered. Generally speaking this type of patient comes from a home of poor intellect and has been brought up in unhelpful and adverse conditions from which his ideas are formed. Once he has started off on the wrong foot, the difference between his standards and those of society may become greater.

Disciplinary measures adopted by society in order to enforce its will against the asocial and antisocial behaviour of these patients only tend to strengthen his belief that everyone is against him. Society's attempt to impose standards of acceptable behaviour is misunderstood because of his many unhappy experiences and his inability to learn from past experience. He repeats the same offences time after time and each succeeding punishment is more severe and the patient becomes more antisocial.

It is not possible to change the subnormal's personality or intelligence. However, it is possible to bring about a change of attitude and outlook. The psychopathically disordered patient does not like being in constant trouble and would, if he were able, stop his bad behaviour.

The patient has no respect for those people who allow him to get away with his waywardness, but prefers those who exercise discipline because this gives him a feeling of security in knowing where he stands.

A healthy stable environment is essential and it is important that the nurse realizes that she forms a part of the environment, and that this environment is responsible for the major proportion of effective treatment and training.

There are many occasions when these patients need advice and guidance. In some cases the advice of a specialist, such as a psychiatrist or psychologist, is needed. Mostly, however, it is the nurse who is able to assist with everyday problems and to offer sympathy and understanding.

Temporary disturbances leading to impulsive actions and outbursts of temper often occur and may be caused by a misunderstanding of relationship or due to not receiving letters from home. If a good and warm relationship exists between the nurse and patient it is usually possible to tackle these problems before they become disciplinary disturbances.

Unfortunately for the nurse the patient may not come to her with his problems. He does not often realize that he has problems. If he does, he does not realize that they can be solved. He may imagine that he has not had a fair deal and has been neglected because of his mental subnormality. The emotions build up within the patient causing outbursts of moodiness and strained relationships and if not noticed and treated as soon as these symptoms appear, more spectacular behaviour such as absenting himself from the hospital and aggressive outbursts towards other patients and staff will occur. Prevention is better than cure, it therefore behoves the nurse to be on the look-out for the slightest change in the patient's behaviour and relationships.

PROGNOSIS

The influence of the environment in augmenting or minimizing the child's mental handicap and the capacity of the human beings associated with him to make the most of his potentials will greatly influence the prognosis.

A mentally subnormal child brought up in a family in which the parents play with him and stimulate his motor development will be much less retarded than the child who is left without maternal attention.

Maternal attention and training will make an enormous difference to the rate at which subnormal children will develop. They will thrive on patient, repetitive training and, if steadily pressed by their parents, will learn to do things which, if left to themselves, would be outside their compass.

One of the difficulties in estimating the potential prognosis is in estimating to what extent environmental factors at the time of diagnosis have stimulated the child to act at his optimal capacity.

Very often the parents' anxiety and self-criticism will result in their rejection of the child and adversely affect the prognosis. It is often common for the rejection to take the form of general neglect and apathy, a feeling that nothing can be done and that the subnormal child must take his chance along with everybody else. This is particularly true of the attitude among the so-called ' social problem families ' who are incapable of effective action.

Among families with a better social status rejection may be replaced by over-compensation. This can take the forms of denying that the child is mentally subnormal or of the parents accepting the diagnosis and, by their will-power and domination, trying to prove the doctors wrong, only to cause the child's prognosis to be worse instead of better.

Prior to recent years mental subnormality was considered hopeless and beyond man's efforts to help ; therefore, as far as treatment and training were concerned, the patient was neglected. Nowadays, the training of the mentally subnormal person is occupying more and more of the civilized nations' efforts. It has now become apparent that very few mentally subnormal people are beyond help, even though in some cases improvement can only be made in the areas of habit training and cleanliness, and in the curtailment of destructive and dangerous propensities. It is now thought possible in some cases to effect a cure if diagnosed early enough.

CHAPTER VII

EDUCATION OF THE MENTALLY SUBNORMAL

THE teacher of the mentally subnormal child has a primary function of establishing a relationship with the child so that together they may widen the boundaries of the child's knowledge, skills, and attitudes. This is not an easy task, for in addition to extending the child's intellectual horizons, there is the continuous need of teaching and reinforcing basic personal skills that are usually taken for granted. The important quality of the teacher is her ability to identify with the child so that she may know when to proffer a new experience, when to assist in interpreting situations, and when to suggest ways of coping with conflicting drives. An important asset is the community which both teacher and child may call upon for assisting in the learning situation. As in a normal adult–child relationship the teacher must indicate the limits of freedom and exercise judgement in allocating responsibility to the child and she must find ways of disciplining and promoting independence without straining relationships.

The teacher has to be able to offer supportive counselling, interpreting diverse attitudes and giving encouragement when failure threatens the security of the child.

In the education of the mentally subnormal person, the activities performed by him must satisfy his needs, desires, and capacities. Where there is severe intellectual limitations it is thought to be a waste of time to teach skills which cannot be put to a practical use; formal training for these children therefore has no real value but should be replaced by training and developing skills and abilities which are meaningful to the child and which will be useful to him in his limited world. It is possible and useful to teach him words which he is likely to meet with frequently and also to make him familiar with coins in common use.

It is useful to teach him to recognize the printed words denoting place names, land-marks, street names, and bus destinations. Recognition of common signs is important, such as, Danger, Ladies, Gentlemen, No Smoking, Entrance, Exit, Keep Out, Poison, Stop, etc.

The attention span of the mentally subnormal person is very short, and in order to learn he must pay attention to all sensory impulses, using a series of games and exercises to develop the special senses of sight, hearing, touch, taste, and smell. Subnormal patients cannot achieve the skills and degrees in knowledge of the three Rs, i.e., reading, writing, and arithmetic, attained by the average child ; therefore the teacher's aims should be :—

1. To train the patient in the art of getting along with his fellow men—social competency can be gained through social experiences.

2. To train him in the habits of work for the purpose of earning his own living. Occupational competence will only result through efficient vocational guidance and training as part of the school curriculum.

3. To help him to develop emotional security and independence in the school and home through a good, affectionate, mental hygiene programme.

4. To develop hygienic and clean habits through health education.

5. To teach the patient how to occupy and enjoy his leisure time through a programme of recreational and leisure-time activities.

6. To aim at making him an adequate member of the family group through a programme emphasizing home membership.

7. To aim at making him an adequate member of the community by emphasis in education on community participation.

The methods of obtaining these aims can be summarized as follows :—

Occupational Adequacy.—The mentally subnormal person should be trained in such a way that he will be able to support himself either wholly or partially. The work he will be most successful in will be unskilled and semi-skilled activities. The patient's success in his job is going to depend upon his getting to work on time, his personal appearance, manners, and health, his ability to get along with other employees and his employer, ability to handle money wisely, safety on the job, and responsibility in following directions and carrying out a task to completion.

The school teacher should from the beginning aim at developing a responsible, efficient worker, regardless of how unskilled the job is. Reading, writing, and arithmetic are part of the occupational education, as the patient will require a minimum of these skills in order to be independent.

Social Adequacy.—The mentally subnormal person should be taught how to get along with his fellow men in a co-operative relationship. He should be educated in how to co-operate with other people at work and play, and be encouraged to show consideration for the rights and desires of other people. This training should begin as soon as the patient enters a school for the mentally subnormal and continue until he leaves to become a stable member of the community.

Personal Adequacy.—The patient must be imbued with a feeling of security within his group and a feeling of belonging. A mentally subnormal person, like a normal child, will have his security shattered if he is unable to compete with others in his group in the school curriculum. Every patient must gain his own self-respect, and the best way of achieving this is through the ability to accomplish something which to him is worth while. Taking an active part in clubs, Scouts, etc., will help the patient to reach a sense of personal happiness and security.

EDUCATION OF THE YOUNG MENTALLY SUBNORMAL CHILD

The mentally subnormal child must be taught all things which will make him socially acceptable. Normal children will absorb much of this basic behaviour from their school companions and their home surroundings without specific teaching. To a subnormal person it must all be taught. The nurse must keep herself aware of what is expected of the child in the community and encourage such standards in the ward and at play.

Cuddling and mothering of patients will bring about a significant decrease in asocial behaviour and purposeless activity. Even the more severely disordered patient will under a 'mother love' condition be stimulated to more purposeful activity to such a degree that the most optimistic nurse will be surprised. Most patients experiencing this love will have a desire to share these experiences with others. They will engage in more social and communicative efforts and, where speech ability is possible, verbal experience will develop.

One of the greatest handicaps from which our patients suffer, in particular the severely subnormal patient, is the poor experience of verbal sensation. Studies of speech development with the normal child have outlined the importance of positive verbal reinforcement from the adult. The child can only develop a meaningful vocabulary to the extent of the opportunity to hear the spoken word. Language development will only occur in a stimulating environment.

It is important, therefore, that we do not deprive our patients of this normal stimulation. Every opportunity to provide verbal stimulation should be taken.

The sense of touch and muscular sense are best taught through actually handling objects of varying sizes, shapes, degrees of smoothness, temperature, and weight. Only through contact with the sensory stimuli will experience of them be gained and be available for recall at a later date. Young patients will find greater opportunity for the expression of their mental life in play and creative activity, and this form of expression persists in the skill of the older child and adult. Therefore, if the patient possesses only one skill this should be used to provide the stimulus for the need to create. The general aim should be to work towards the socialization of the patient, to give him creative outlets for the use of his intelligence, to supply healthy outlets for his normal aggressive feeling, and to re-establish self-confidence. To achieve this it will be necessary to have a planned programme in which each activity has a goal, never prolonged so that it becomes boring, and to have a kind, firm discipline which ensures that every child is occupied and every child is respected as being an important individual. The nurse should talk to each of the children in her care with the politeness and good manners that she expects them to learn, and she should adopt an attitude of patience and understanding during tantrum disturbances which are bound to arise from time to time. In this way the child will absorb and adopt acceptable standards. The patient is thus treated as if he were a normal child, with allowance being made for his handicap. A subnormal person has a dignity belonging to his chronological age-group.

Unless the nurse can experience a broad and real sense of love for her patients and her work, which are the essence of her dedicated vocation, the work will be impossible.

No time is lost when the subnormal child first arrives at the hospital. He is introduced to his group, which should be a small one, with whom he is to live and work, and from the beginning he is encouraged to help others, to share with them, and to think beyond himself.

The basic social needs are made the subject of strict routine at the outset, and this in itself will quickly influence his whole attitude to the hospital. The basic subjects are : (1) Personal cleanliness : (2) Toilet routine ; (3) Table manners ; (4) Social adequacy ; (5) Tidiness and personal appearance, care of clothes ; (6) Posture.

Personal cleanliness does not come naturally in subnormals, and it is of first importance that they should wash before meals, after going to the lavatory, and when they are dirty, with such regularity that they feel it is part of the action itself. In this way they are conditioned to be clean, and the behaviour pattern may become fixed so that it will remain with them all their lives. As in everything else they must be shown how to wash and dry themselves in detail again and again so that the technique is learned and overlearned. Bathing should be taught in the same way, the child being encouraged to perform the task himself and not expecting to be treated as a baby.

This will require repetition for many years, but it must be taught.

Toilet routine must be regular, sufficiently frequent, and quite matter of fact. As a practical matter, it is an excellent rule that whichever member of the staff notices a child to have been incontinent should immediately deal with it. It is a disagreeable duty, but, shared equally by the whole staff, it can be dealt with in a matter-of-fact way to the benefit of the child and the morale of the staff.

Table manners are very essential for the child if he is to be able to feel that he is a person acceptable to society. At first the child should be shown repeatedly how to use a spoon and fork and later a knife. He is taught to say ' please ' and ' thank you ', or, if he has no speech, to give and take things gently. One means of teaching them service to others is to allow the children to take it in turns to wait on the other patients at table, to lay the table for meals, and to clear the table after meals.

Social manners, like all other aspects of training, begin on the very first day of admission, and continue throughout the whole period in hospital. Like everything else they are taught over and over again until they become the child's normal responses to particular situations.

The teaching will include : shaking hands, closing doors on entering or leaving a room, being introduced and introducing, gentlemen standing until ladies are seated, opening the door for visitors, putting away his own equipment, tidying up the recreation room for the next users.

With increasing age, lessons will be given in accepting greater responsibility, such as shopping and the use and value of money, travelling and behaviour in public transport, using public lavatories, road sense and the use of zebra crossings, time and punctuality.

From his social training within the hospital the child will get the idea of helping others in everyday situations.

Personal tidiness, care of clothes, and the importance of his appearance are all important. If an element of competition is introduced and frequent inspections are made the teaching will be all the more successful and will create less friction.

Posture is of importance as the ill-trained patient is often conspicuous in the community due to his slouching gait.

The nurse must approach her part as teacher with the idea firmly fixed in her mind that all children are capable of being taught something and that none of her efforts will be wasted. The lessons will begin at any age, continuing into adult life, and through this teaching the patient will gain the idea of self, the satisfaction of being of service to others, and of being accepted by others.

EDUCATION OF THE OLDER MENTALLY SUBNORMAL PERSON

The curriculum for these patients should be an extension of that for the younger mentally subnormal person and the objectives the same.

Academic subjects should be of secondary importance, but all those able to benefit from the training should receive instruction in the three Rs to the level of their mental ability. When teaching reading and writing it is important to ensure that comprehension of meaning keeps pace with the ability to read mechanically.

The teaching of writing and spelling should be carried out in relation to other school activities and experiences. Lists of equipment can be made by the patients for their next classes, and descriptive stories giving an account of their experiences while out walking can be used as writing aids. Accuracy and legibility should not be neglected for speed, which should never be regarded as important. Accidental approaches will not develop if the correct position and procedure for writing are taught and practised from the outset. Writing must have meaning to the subnormal, and correlation between writing, reading, and spelling will help in this.

Art, whether in the form of music, drawing, or painting, is a means of expression and has no confining limits in age, ability, or capability. It is usually in arts and crafts that the mentally subnormal person finds his greatest satisfaction. Art can be used to illustrate stories and rhymes ; watching his work grow and take shape increases his interest and attention.

The easiest and most successful way of promoting interest in crafts is to allow the subnormal to choose his own project. An attitude of pride in the work carried out should be encouraged and this can be done by allowing him to keep and use objects he has made. The shared use of equipment, the care of tools, and the leaving of tools so that others can find them and use them, all help in preparing the patient for social living.

The activities in the class-room, the attitude of the teacher towards the patient, and the curriculum, each has a bearing upon the patient's personality development and his behaviour in and out of school. A busy and interesting class-room will offer very little time for misbehaviour. The work should be planned beforehand, so that the children are in a learning situation all the time and doing something that is interesting. The teacher should encourage the patient to solve his own problems even though it allows of making mistakes. Behaviour is determined to a great extent by the group's approval, and when the group has defined its own rules of conduct the individuals are more apt to abide by them.

Behaviour, whether it be good behaviour or misbehaviour, is a means of adjustment. Whatever the patient does is a means of attempting to reduce tension. If the teacher and the nurse understand this they will find it easier to make adjustments when necessary in the patient's activities.

EDUCATION OF THE SEVERELY SUBNORMAL

In hospitals today the emphasis is strongly on the admission of the severely subnormal patient and the provision of community care for the stable mentally subnormal. The severely subnormal patient has a greater need of the services of the conscientious nurse for care and training than has any other class of patient. The system of training given must be constant throughout the whole of the patients' lives otherwise they will deteriorate and lose what initiative they have gained. Many of them are admitted to hospital as bedridden patients, unable to attempt the simplest co-ordinated motor movements.

Cripples can be taught how to walk, in many cases, by encouraging them to walk between parallel bars. Toys placed slightly out of reach will also stimulate movement. Most bed- and chair-ridden patients should be able to take exercise, provided the muscles of their legs and arms are strengthened. Even with an adequate physiotherapy department, progress will only be maintained by the daily efforts of the nurse on the ward. If physical exercise classes have a background of music the desire to move will be stimulated. The use of solid, strong equipment to assist movement is necessary as an aid to walking and will be needed by many patients. The pattern of the equipment can be similar to that used by the average small child, provided it is strong and large enough to support the weight of the patient. Exercises should be limited to set periods each day so that the patient does not become stale and his deformed limbs fatigued.

Elementary sensory training is provided through the use of peg boards, nests of cubes and boxes, sets of buttons and button-holes, sets of simple picture puzzles, and paper to cut. The first steps in stitching can be taken, the patient trying to thread a blunt needle with bright coloured thread through holes bored in a piece of wood. Simple occupations can be taught, such as wood bundling, boot cleaning, polishing brass and cutlery, and simple household and personal duties. When training the severely subnormal, spectacular and rapid results should not be expected, but ultimately social self-respect, happiness, and independence will replace apathy, discontentment, and destructive habits.

THE EDUCATION OF THE DEAF CHILD

Deafness is not only a handicap of not being able to hear; in children with severe hearing loss it is a barrier to hearing speech, the normal means of communication accepted by society. Words are sound symbols representing objects, ideas, and feelings. Apart from enabling us to communicate with others, they aid us in thinking, in storing knowledge, and in formulating concepts. In being unable to hear the words his mother speaks to him a deaf child is deprived of learning language and speech. It is essential for a deaf child to learn to speak, to learn language, to learn to lip-read others' speech so that he can lead a normal life.

The true meaning of education is the development of a person spiritually, morally, mentally, and physically. Education is not the prerogative of schools, it is concerned with the home (in the case of a child in hospital with his ward) and society. We are all mutually involved in educating each other throughout our lives. The education of the child, therefore, is not just the responsibility of the teachers, it is the responsibility of his parents, relations, and all people who come into contact with him.

The role which the parent and nurse of deaf and partially hearing children play in the education of their children is especially important, since these children have to learn language and speech without the facility of hearing.

A stimulating environment will prompt children to think and ask questions about their environment. From the answers they receive they acquire a vast amount of knowledge. These children need the same number of opportunities to develop an inquiring mind and to learn about their environment as do normal-hearing children. In addition, they need to develop special skills such as lip-reading, acquiring language and speech without the natural faculty of hearing in order to do this.

A hearing-aid will only be efficiently used if the microphone of the aid is placed within a foot of the wearer's mouth and if the speaker stands within a foot of the child, the child will then hear his own speech and that of other people with the maximum amplification. Since the speech the child hears through his hearing-aid will be distorted, his own speech will also be distorted; in order to supplement this he will have to depend on the efficient use of his hearing-aid, the lip-reading of consonants on people's mouths, and on being taught how to produce consonants properly.

Lip-reading depends upon having some idea of the subject matter.

Normal children acquire language by hearing words repeated in meaningful situations many times throughout life. Deaf children can learn language in the same manner provided that they make use of their residual hearing and of lip-reading, and that they can see the object referred to or an illustration of it.

The nurse should develop a talking environment in the ward, talking naturally, distinctly, and often to the child. Normal activities, such as dressing and undressing the child, give the nurse the opportunity of holding up an article of clothing and repeating its name in a natural sentence. At first the nurse will find it requires a great deal of effort ; however, given time, the development of a talking environment will become second nature to the nurse and the child, and other residents of the ward and staff.

The nurse should first of all encourage the child to babble and vocalize. This can be achieved by holding a balloon between his hands and resting it on his lips and then babbling on to it. He will feel the vibrations and he should then be encouraged to try to make the same vibrations until the babbling becomes speech.

A high-powered hearing-aid is available which has greater amplification over speech frequencies, and speech is reproduced better through it than through an ordinary wearable hearing-aid.

SPEECH TRAINING

Whatever the cause of the defect of speech in a mentally subnormal patient, every effort must be made to stimulate the use of the vocal cords. In the first place, the speech therapist and the nurse must be quite certain that the patient is not deaf, and, secondly, must not ignore a patient who is unable to speak, but encourage him to watch others talking and to listen.

Lack of stimulus for speech is one of the serious environmental defects of a hospital for the mentally subnormal. The speech therapist must endeavour to create a need for speech and help the child to build up his vocabularly to meet his needs. Praise and encouragement should be given liberally.

Most interest and research are being directed towards the care of the cerebrally palsied child.

The first aim in treatment must be to establish correct feeding habits as far as possible and to correct head and neck posture and movements of respiration in the early stages of treatment.

The patient must be encouraged to relax completely and then be allowed to babble vocally so that he can experience some of the sensations of normal effortless speech.

It is not uncommon for the speech therapist to work in conjunction with the physiotherapist and occupational therapist.

Occasionally a patient is discovered who has an inability to appreciate the meaning of spoken words with the absence of, or marked defect of, speech. The child is not severely deaf; he can hear many of the common sounds. Because of the uncertainty of the possible site of defect, progress in the diagnosis and treatment is very slow. Loss of certain frequencies of hearing will give children ' islands of hearing ' without the ability to discriminate between the sounds used in human speech.

Any doubtful cases should be seen and tested by the audio-metrician who has specialized amplification equipment which tests the hearing at various frequencies, following which the patient should be seen by an E.N.T. specialist for medical advice and treatment.

Patients with defective hearing may be helped by the use of a hearing aid. Many of the earlier difficulties of selective amplification at the affective frequencies are being overcome. The pattern of the aids is being modernized to a less cumbersome and lighter style.

In creating speech impressions for the patient the nurse must speak very deliberately and slowly, and must make full use of the lips as one would do for any young child. Articles of common usage and interest should be pointed out and named repeatedly. Speech training through the stimulus of playing games will make the patient want to speak and encourage him to make the effort. Once speech has begun to develop and progress, reading lessons should begin, the nurse using pictures as aids.

Flannel-graphs are a simple form of visual aid in which the blackboard is replaced by a lint-covered board and the chalk by paper letters and pictures. Pads of lint are attached to the back of the picture or word and are easily adherent to the lint-covered board. As the teacher tells her story, she graphically illustrates it by applying an appropriate word and picture to the board and by this means the relationship of words and objects can be built up.

RELIGIOUS MINISTRY TO THE MENTALLY SUBNORMAL

In the hospital caring for the mentally subnormal patient, emphasis should be placed on the provision of the services of a chaplain to cover the Church of England, Roman Catholic, and Nonconformist denominations.

The chaplains should be more than 'Conductors of Services'; they should be every patient's confidant and friend.

It is important that the chaplain be accepted as one of the hospital's team, as he, with the other members, is striving for the same end. The nurse should give her fullest co-operation to him. Effective religious care demands this for an atmosphere of friendliness and devotion. The nurse, it must be remembered, is well acquainted with the patient's needs.

Opportunity should be offered for private interviews with the patient, especially with new admissions, so that a link between the patient's home and church can be maintained.

The work of the chaplain will be focused on the patient and the world he lives in day after day, and his services are there for all to enjoy irrespective of their mental and physical state.

Göte Bergston in his *Pastoral Psychology* has set forth the pastor's work thus :—

1. Healing through forgiveness, reconciliation, and faith.
2. Instruction or re-education.
3. Guidance in practical matters.

Religious care means removing fears, substituting right for wrong ideas, and inculcating a positive attitude to life.

Opportunity should be provided for the chaplain and the nurse to discuss the individual patients and their problems, and between them come to some suitable solution.

It must be remembered that the nurse and chaplain are two people who are students of their own individual calling, and that where the needs of an individual person require the services of two such people, some form of mutual consultation should take place to give the patient the benefit of a combined effort.

8

The teaching of the Christian way of life should not only come from the chaplain but he should also prepare the foundation for such teaching and the nurse should assist with the building up of a Christian life upon that foundation.

Mentally subnormal patients are good imitators, and what the nursing staff say and the way they behave today the patient will follow tomorrow. The nurse's life should therefore be beyond reproach and her conduct of benefit to the patient.

Whilst the mentally subnormal has many physical needs, he also has spiritual needs which can best be met through religious instruction, provided through a trained member of the ministerial profession. Care of the patient which does not include this cannot be considered complete. The mentally subnormal patient is capable of religious devotion. He is usually well behaved at religious services, and takes part in simple devotional services with enjoyment.

There is no doubt that religion gives these patients a richer life and a code of living which they would not have otherwise. They learn to express their thoughts through prayer, and welcome the opportunity to join a congregation in worship.

The chaplain is the only member of the staff who can give patients concrete hope for the future.

Physical health is not the primary object in dealing with a mentally subnormal patient, but rather his general well-being. The medical staff, the nursing staff, the chaplain, and all the other members of the hospital staff each has his own particular function, and through them the whole of the patient's personality is catered for—that is, his body, mind, and spirit. Without harmonious working of all these three, his health and well-being can never be achieved.

HABIT TRAINING

By habit training is meant the utilization of energy towards carrying out desired and essential activities, such as eating, urinating, and sleeping, in the right manner and at the correct time.

Through a regular routine of life, it is hoped to appeal to the patient's senses and thus to stimulate interest in life and provide opportunity for spontaneity.

Owing to his affection for the nurse the child will gradually show signs of improvement even though he has no particular desire to improve. Every stage must be gained by affection and with the child's consent for the cure to be of a permanent nature.

As in the training of normal children, obedience is absolutely essential. The training must be performed painlessly—in other words, the patient must be educated to the fact that to obey is kinder to himself and to those who love him.

In the case of a mentally subnormal person, reasoning power cannot give us aid in our teaching. His problems must be thought out and solutions provided.

In the teaching process, each stage can be performed as a game which stimulates interest. Attention must be concentrated entirely on teaching. If a command is issued one must see that it is carried out successfully and show interest in the end-result.

The patient's day should be so full, varied, and interesting that his bad habits are crowded out of his life. Bad habits are usually a result of an unoccupied mind finding an outlet for its energy.

Health and comfort of the body are indispensable as a sound foundation upon which to work. Any ill health or discomfort will cause disturbance of the mind to such a degree that the patient will mutilate himself, and adopt aggressive and destructive habits to attract the attention of those around. Therefore a healthy, comfortable body will produce a peace of mind conducive to the reception of training.

It is important here to remember that all mentally subnormal people are really children, no matter what their age. Normal children up to eighteen months receive pleasure from contact with their warm, wet excretions. It is therefore to be expected that subnormal persons will receive similar pleasure, only more so, and will be less responsive to training.

The habits of mentally subnormal patients are usually dirty, and unless they are taught good clean habits, through training and example, their condition will deteriorate. They can be educated to an appreciation of their own personal hygiene and a clean healthy environment. If unhygienic conditions prevail flies are attracted which torment the patient and cause him hours of misery. Patients must develop the habit of cleanliness, and it is a task that demands great skill, patience, and dogged perseverance on the part of the nursing staff.

There are patients who have the habit of emptying their bladders so frequently that the stream never appears to stop. Such patients require attention at least every ten minutes; after meals the time should be shortened to five minutes. The training must continue during the night as well as the day, and for the first two hours in bed the patient should be attended to every fifteen minutes, and every thirty minutes for the next hour and a half. Then once in the next hour, and once in the following two hours. He should remain clean from 2 a.m. until waking, although it may be found that some patients will require attention between these times. With constant attention and training, results can be expected which will astound all who know the patient. It is in fact possible to render most patients completely independent and able to retain their evacuation for normal periods. However, accidents will occur, particularly during illness, to the great consternation of the patient himself. The nurse must be prepared to take this in her stride and avoid drawing undue attention to it.

It is possible for nurses to be so 'incontinence conscious' that they overlook the fact that it is possible for patients to suffer from a retention of urine with or without overflow. Only strict observation and an inquiring mind will detect that this condition is present. It can have serious consequences and must therefore receive immediate attention.

It is more difficult to train a patient in bowel control than in bladder control. Enemas must be avoided at all costs as these tend to encourage the patient not to try to make an effort. Some authorities advocate the giving of regular but small doses of aperient (large doses do not encourage the patient to make an effort) to help form a bowel habit. Regular opportunity for bowel action must be offered in ideal conditions—a well-lighted toilet, comfortable seating, and a warm environment.

Children or older patients who have many bowel actions in a day are usually very hungry and at meal times tend to bolt their food, resulting, in many cases, in digestive disturbances ; and although these may be treated with a mild alkaline mixture they are better dealt with by persuading and encouraging the patient to eat more slowly.

The same preparations for meals should be made for the patients as for normal people. Conversation should be allowed during meal times, the patients being encouraged to talk about the day's occupations. Pauses between courses are essential as digestive aids. Every effort should be made to educate the patients to feed themselves. Their clothing must be protected as it must be expected that they will make a mess in their early endeavours. Much time and patience will be required before results will show, but little is to be gained by the nurse weakening in her teaching and feeding the patient herself.

The diet will require the co-operation of the nursing staff, the dietitian, and the kitchen staff. All are responsible for seeing that there is a variety of food, that it is properly prepared and cooked, and if intended to be hot, served hot, and in an appetizing manner. Any food the nurse considers unsuitable should be returned to the kitchen.

The cause of any patient refusing food should be investigated immediately ; it may only be because of not feeling hungry, but it may be caused by an oncoming illness which may be aborted by early medical attention.

Most people have some bad habits which form part of their lives, but usually they are so insignificant as to cause no distress. If a patient's mind becomes unoccupied it will find employment in unhealthy habits such as nail biting, flesh picking, or aggressive behaviour. Exercise which demands voluntary effort will replace this form of occupation. All unoccupied moments must be utilized to good purpose to encourage the patient in social habits.

Personal toilet is an activity which every individual should be encouraged to attend to personally, but under supervision. Each patient should be taught to attend to cleaning his own teeth and to washing. To stimulate the desire to do it himself, each washing session should be a game in which each patient has a part. Encouragement and guidance will be needed by the patient, and patience by the nurse. The wash-bowls should be of a suitable height so that the patients can wash conveniently. A washing time-table should be prepared and adhered to. By example hand washing should be taught after each visit to the toilet, and before each meal; and a thorough washing of hands and face on waking in the morning, and if a daily bath is impracticable, before retiring to bed at night.

Most patients can be taught to dress themselves quite adequately, provided that the training is carried out slowly and only one stage at a time is taught; two stages are overpowering and they cannot cope. Buttons and button-holes should be large and easy to manipulate because the mentally subnormal person has not got the same suppleness, muscle control, and dexterity as a normal child and so finds it difficult to handle small objects.

Bed-time should be early to ensure that the patients have adequate rest. Warm baths should be given before retiring, if possible, as these are both relaxing and sedative in their action, qualities which will benefit all patients. All the excitement of a game can be put into the bathing, thus gaining the patient's co-operation.

It must be stressed that the perfection of a normal mind is not to be expected of a mentally subnormal person, but rather perfections of their own capabilities. Too much must not be expected, neither must too little. The struggle to overcome difficulties will add to the desire in most patients to learn and become self-sufficient. The aspirations, then, of the nurse must not exceed the capacity of the patient.

Praise and reward will promote efficiency and contentment where reproof and punishment would produce disturbed behaviour. Patience, tolerance, reasonableness, fairness, and consistency are the keynotes to success.

The more severely subnormal patient will be found to be less responsive to training. Even so, he will have potentialities which will have to be cultivated or made use of. It is possible to render most patients clean and dry by a system of repetitive training which must be regular. Because results do not appear to be forthcoming, it must not be assumed that complete failure will be the outcome—results *can* be expected, if not immediately. The nurse's degree of expectancy must inevitably be less than for the subnormal patient. More patience will be required and dogged perseverance. Love and affection are important factors ; the lowest loves recognition, and will respond to it.

The observant nurse will recognize three temperamental groups amongst her patients :—

1. The Facile.—The patient is easily led and very responsive to suggestion.

2. The Apathetic.—These patients have a placid disposition, are rarely in trouble, and are good workers, but they lack initiative.

3. The Unstable.—This type of patient is bad-tempered. His work is spasmodic and unreliable, but very occasionally he shows initiative.

The first two groups will respond quite happily to their training, which they are usually physically able to carry out, together with all forms of activities, and as a rule they cause very little trouble. Their potentialities are such that great improvement can be expected and so long as training is constant, improvement will continue. These patients should be completely self-sufficient and only require supervision.

The third group, the unstable, must be led rather than driven and encouraged when they fail.

All hospitals for the mentally subnormal have born leaders amongst their patients. These can be trained to act as prefects and leaders of a group, but they will require close supervision by the nursing staff to see that no unfair treatment occurs.

DELINQUENCY

The definition of delinquency is ' antisocial behaviour '. The individual, in spite of accepting all that society can offer, refuses to conform to the standards set by society and resorts to a life of vice and crime. A combination of antisocial behaviour and low intelligence will produce a person at present described as mentally subnormal, and someone likely to require care and training in hospital.

Most mentally subnormal people are harmless, inoffensive, tractable, and well-conducted members of society. They differ from the normal in their want of common sense and full understanding. Others are not only subnormal, they are also prone to misconduct, and this is often so vicious, or criminal, as to cause them to be a serious social danger, and therefore is likely to require hospitalization over a long period.

The cause, as well as the type, of antisocial behaviour varies in different individuals. Delinquency of differing levels of intelligence has been classified as follows: (1) Benign, (2) Temperamental, (3) Simple, (4) Reactionary.

1. Benign Delinquency.—Often children with adventurous spirits commit misdemeanours which occasionally bring them before the Magistrates, though the crime will not have been committed with intent to offend or do harm, but rather as an outlet for their adventurous natures. In some it is due to a want of understanding that their acts are wrong.

2. Temperamental Delinquency.—Changes in the physiological functions will cause an otherwise respectable person to commit crimes. Physiological changes in girls and women frequently cause a loss of balance which allows them to give way to their impulses.

3. Simple Delinquency.—These children are the product of environmental impulses, for example, poverty, overcrowding, drunkenness, and prostitution in the home, bad upbringing such as spoiling, too strict upbringing, lack of discipline, wrong type of discipline, bad parents, and bad companions.

4. Reactionary Delinquency.—This condition is caused by the child being brought up in an environment in which he is denied the love and affection which all children so badly need, as a result of which complexes are formed which determine his behaviour. Consciousness of his defect, or of being different, may itself be responsible for feelings of inferiority, frustration, and resentment in the case of some subnormals, which may cause them to commit acts of violent aggressiveness and destructiveness which are unconsciously directed towards self-assertiveness.

THE EDUCATIONALLY SUBNORMAL CHILD

These children vary in degree of retardation and possess an I.Q. of 70 or less. Because of their serious degree of retardation they cannot be taught satisfactorily in ordinary classes or schools. Their education is carried out under the direction of the Education Act, 1944, which made the provision of special schools compulsory.

Though these children possess the I.Q. of the subnormal person they do differ from the subnormal in that they can adapt themselves to the requirements of society and are capable of a high degree of self-care.

Dull and Backward Children.—Though these two types of children are classed together they nevertheless are different in degree and cause of retardation. Both conditions also vary in their response to treatment.

Dull Children.—The cause of dullness is innate. It is a condition characterized by an all-round mental inferiority. Learning is difficult, memory, logical thinking, and reasoning are poor, and the child has difficulty with any subject that is abstract.

The emotional instability and intellectual inferiority of these children may enhance the occurrence of delinquency and render them in need of care, supervision, and control.

Backward Children.—This condition is due to external causes and the degree of retardation is not so severe as in the dull child. If the causes were removed the condition would revert to normal.

The causes of backwardness may be classified as : (1) Environmental ; (2) Physical ; (3) Slow development.

1. *Environmental causes* : Poor home conditions where there is a poverty of teaching stimuli and loss of security within its confines ; irregular attendance at school and frequent changes of school ; faulty teaching techniques and harsh methods of teaching.

2. *Physical causes* : Defectiveness of the special senses of sight, hearing, and speech ; illness due to enlarged tonsils and

adenoids; malnutrition; inadequate sleep and rest; chronic diseases such as heart disease, rheumatic fever, and tuberculosis; epilepsy.

3. *Slow development* : Some children are backward because they do not mentally mature along the normal lines, some maturing too late to benefit from normal school education. The cause of this is unknown.

The dull and the backward child both need individual teaching of a specialized form from specially qualified teachers.

Whereas the dull child will remain dull and progress very little, the backward child will advance towards normal.

Special Schools for Educationally Subnormal Children.—Special schools may be residential or day schools. The larger educational authorities have need of their own special schools and the children are day attenders. For the smaller authorities whose need is only for a few places, residential schools are made available where children from several authorities may be housed and given special teaching.

The aim of the special school is to make of the educationally subnormal child an efficient citizen, self respecting and self supporting as far as possible, and socially acceptable in his habits.

The education given is practical, concrete, and vocational. The three Rs are only taught to the level necessary for everyday social intercourse—how to read direction notices, warnings of danger, how to handle money to avoid being cheated. Clear speech is an advantage to the child, therefore great care is taken in teaching clear enunciation.

Educationally subnormal children attend school until they attain the age of 16 years. They are medically examined at yearly intervals and any change in their physical and emotional condition is noted.

CHILD GUIDANCE CLINICS

Child guidance clinics are for the treatment of behaviour problems in nervous, unstable, and difficult children. Their aim is to prevent adult neuroses by attention to mental hygiene. While they rarely treat mentally subnormal children, nevertheless many subnormal children are unstable, and for this reason some knowledge of the work of such a clinic, with possibly a visit to see one in action, is necessary.

Cases are referred to the clinics by family doctors, school medical officers, teachers, parents, children's courts, and child care committees. The difficulties include those of nervousness, backwardness at school, and lack of adjustment to home or school, which, if not dealt with, might lead to delinquency. Some of the commonest causes for referring a child to the clinic are bed-wetting, sex difficulties, truancy, theft, temper, and night terrors.

The staff of a child guidance clinic consists of a psychiatrist, an educational psychologist, and a psychiatric social worker. The psychiatrist carries out the physical and general mental examination. The educational psychologist assesses the attainments and the development of the child by interview and intelligence testing. The psychiatric social worker investigates the home environment. Home visits are made before and after treatment and efforts are made to persuade the parents to make some adjustment in the child's régime which will help to solve his behaviour difficulties.

Play Therapy.—Play therapy has two important assets : (1) The value of play therapy as a diagnostic aid ; (2) The value of play therapy as a form of treatment and training for the unemployable severely subnormal person.

1. *The value of play therapy as a diagnostic aid* : In this way a diagnosis may be made or treatment carried out. Most children express and resolve their emotional difficulties through their play. A child will, for instance, play at being a soldier because the soldier seems strong and important in contrast to his own weakness and dependence.

In the clinic playroom, children are supplied with a variety of toys which include sand, water, blackboard and chalk, a doll's house, model figures, animals, trains, and motor-cars. They are left to do what they like with them, while skilled observers make records of what the children do. As a result of the clinic's investigation, advice may be given as to more consistent treatment at home, or less stern and repressive discipline, or recommendation for a change of school.

2. *The value of play therapy as a form of treatment and training for the unemployable severely subnormal person* : At the outset, it is important that there exists a good relationship between the nurse and patient, that his needs and desires are satisfied, and that his own individuality is recognized. The aim must always be to find and develop the patient's hidden potentials.

When viewing a class of 30 severely subnormals, the nurse should see them as 30 individuals, each being different from every other member of his group, and requiring a diversity of approaches. Every one of these patients is attempting to use his limited resources to meet the challenge of his everyday living. The training to be successful should assist the patient to meet the challenge of living more effectively.

Four well-chosen aims should be used as a guide to those responsible for the training of the severely subnormal : (1) To develop acceptable patterns of personal behaviour ; (2) To develop acceptable patterns of social behaviour ; (3) To develop skills that will make the patient a more useful member of his family and community ; (4) To develop skills that will make him a more contented and useful member of a social group.

When preparing a curriculum for these patients, one must bear in mind the individual, the intelligence quotient of the individual, and the aims. The curriculum should be elastic, in order that it can be moulded to the progress of the patient or be adjusted for the patient who is not showing progress, and that it is developmental in all its aspects. No patient should remain static, movement of learning either forwards and in cases where difficulties are being met, backwards, in order to begin again. Every stage of training must be challenging in order to stimulate learning.

Abstract teaching has little value, therefore all training must be built around real life experience.

The basis of teaching normal children in their primary school days is done through play techniques and it has proved highly successful. The important thing at this stage is keeping in mind the needs of the individual and the needs of the group.

In the management of these patients, it is to be expected that the patient may be unable to communicate, be withdrawn, doubly incontinent, and may have sudden rages.

The curriculum should include prayers and Bible stories, music and movement, toilet training, habit training, speech therapy, relaxation, play and story telling.

A typical daily curriculum as used in the play therapy department at the Brentry Hospital, Bristol, is as follows :—

8.45–9.45 a.m.	Instruction on how to dress, wash, clean teeth, and toilet training.
9.45–10.00	Patients taken to play therapy unit.
10.05–10.15	Prayers and Bible story.
10.15–10.45	Speech therapy. Balance training.
10.45–11.05	Toilet training.
11.05–11.45	Play.
11.45–12 noon	Patients return to their wards for lunch.
12.00–1.15 p.m.	Lunch time.
1.15–2.15	Relaxation.
2.15–2.30	Toilet training and cleaning teeth.
2.30–2.45	Return to play therapy unit.
2.45–3.30	Music and movement.
3.30–4.00	Story telling.
4.00–4.15	Toilet training.
4.15–4.30	Patients return to their wards.

Detailed records of individual progress should be maintained, so that a full and comprehensive picture of each patient is available.

Some patients will develop beyond the play therapy level, and when this happens they should be placed in a more advanced environment, so that their full potential may be reached.

CHAPTER VIII

CARE OF THE MENTALLY SUBNORMAL CHILD

FOR a long time now it has been known that to separate a child from his mother is fraught with danger for the child, hence the aim to keep mentally subnormal children in the home environment during the formative years.

When you are looking after other people's children it is difficult to appreciate the extent to which the child is emotionally involved towards his parents, even though they may have neglected or ill treated him.

By and large hospital care is improving rapidly, but it is possible for babies in hospital nurseries to receive only the minimum of stimulation, diversion, physical contact, physical freedom, and interpersonal contact.

It is important that young children in hospital are placed in the centre of activity so that they can hear and see things moving and they can become aware of any changing stimulus within their environment. Having the patient in such a position in the ward also allows the nurse to notice any change in the patient's condition and to be able to applaud and encourage the child in any effort he may make to move his limbs, sit up, or babble. The child should not be left in one position in his cot for so long that the mattress sinks so much as to prevent him from making any movement. Impersonal care will cause severe blocking of intellectual development.

Sometimes a child who has been in hospital for a long time following early separation appears to forget his parents, but there is a great deal of underlying feeling which may not appear until adolescence, and often in an undesirable manner.

The real importance of the family is continuity of care in which a child develops from one phase to another. This is what children brought up in hospital miss, unless there is a constant person whom the child can hang on to.

The chief damage in separation from home takes place in the early years because at this period of life the parents are the centre of his life.

To mother a child means washing him, cuddling him, putting him on the potty, putting him to bed and getting him up, and making physical contact with him.

When a child is removed from his home and taken into hospital he is put into surroundings which are strange and confusing. It is easy for the nurse to overlook the magnitude of the problem of reorientation, and to forget how much more important things, persons, and places are to a child than to a grown-up. Ordinary everyday objects like his bed, his place at table, his teddy-bear are so closely connected in his mind with the vivid experiences of childhood that they are to him much more than just things, they have the sort of emotional significance which adults usually reserve for people.

Most of the child's learning is active learning ; his experience and his capacity for abstraction are too limited for him to be able to think through complicated problems without engaging in them directly. Any period of inactivity usually causes a temporary slowing down of learning.

The principal danger which attends the separation of the child from his parents is not the sadness and distress of the loss itself, but the fact that he has also lost confidence which has sustained him through all developmental stages. The consequence of this trauma is that the child tends to regress to an infantile level of behaviour.

Often the child deliberately turns his back on the past and shows marked inclination to forget the unpleasant and frightening events. This is his means of coping with a highly stressful situation, and it is tempting to let him go on doing it, but there are good grounds for insisting that this, in the long run, is bad policy ; if he is to grow up into a sound, confident human being, he must come to terms with the events and separation.

At this time the child has three pressing needs, for support, information, and opportunity to act through his traumatic event.

The relationship between the nurse and child must be a warmly affectionate one; it must be genuinely individual and utterly dependable. This is difficult in a hospital ward where there are many more children than nurses, but it is not quite impossible. Perhaps the greatest difficulty is to help a shy and often uncommunicative child to feel that someone in the ward is his own special nurse, that whatever is happening he can always be sure of a warm response from her, even if she has to share her attentions with others.

It is important for the child to be given as much information as possible about his separation from his family and the reasons leading to admission. To adults it may seem that a child must have a perfectly accurate recollection of events but in times of stress most of us tend to be a little stupid, we are so preoccupied with the problem of the moment that we fail to notice elements of the situation which we afterwards realize were important, and we wish that we could recall them.

The opportunity to work through the traumatic events is important. The child tends to learn by doing rather than by abstract thinking. Rehearsing or acting out experiences plays an important part in children's social learning; many childish games are opportunities for arrival at a better understanding of the behaviour of adults by imitating it. Often a child cannot make sense of something his parents have done until he has repeated the incident with the help of other children or of dolls; by acting their parts he can work out for himself what they felt and intended in relation to himself. This technique is often of critical value to a separated child, especially in the form of what is usually called 'testing out behaviour'.

DELINQUENT CHILDREN

When dealing with delinquent children there are two important things which a nurse should practise; they are 'understanding' and 'respect'. This means that the most difficult child must not only meet with understanding but with a deep respect for him as a human being and what he could be. This is not always easy when one is faced with a difficult, aggressive, insolent child. It is only human to feel disappointment, anger, and a desire to retaliate towards those inflicting the pain. The nurse would be helped if she would analyse some of the child's problems and realize that these may be different for each child. Most of us find some difficulty entering a new environment and meeting new people. How much more difficult must it be for a child to be put into this same situation against his wishes and this for an indefinite period. Children are brought into hospital because of difficulty in the family, homes having been broken up, illness or death in the family, domestic strife, or because the child himself is full of emotional problems, or has committed some crime against society.

The tendency in the future will be for the hospitals to take more of the difficult children as patients and less of the easily managed type.

There are many instances where the child's misbehaviour is the result of a lack of order and routine in the home. In some children this creates a sense of insecurity. It is essential, therefore, that the nurse develops an ordered routine which can be understood by each child. Though a disturbed child may find difficulty in leading an orderly life, it is helpful to him to experience a calm and orderly atmosphere. One thing that must be avoided, however, is not to allow the atmosphere to become too rigid.

The problem of the nurse is to know how long to allow untidiness to go unnoticed, or to ignore bad table manners. If the child is pushed he may resent it and his behaviour deteriorate. It is often helpful to sit him next to those who have been in hospital for some little time in order to help him calm down and to demonstrate unobtrusively the correct way to eat and keep himself clean. Slowly, but with occasional reminders, the child will change as his calmness increases.

Sleep is one of the essentials of life and the way the nurse prepares the child for bed can be helpful or harmful to him. Going to bed means much in a child's life. Most children are afraid of the dark at some time. More reassurance is needed therefore in the evening. Getting ready for bed brings a greater opportunity for intimate understanding. In a loving family bedtime is the hour for intimacy between parent and

9

child, there is fun splashing in the bath, having a story read aloud, or just being cuddled. It is not easy for nurses to find time for this kind of understanding, but where the child is denied he will often become disturbed. A few minutes given to each child will give untold rewards.

The need for and importance of privacy is often overlooked, yet it can be the most important need of most patients. Many of the children coming into hospital need help to relate with others and therefore the group situation is very important for them, but they still need the opportunity to get away from the pressure of others ; then there are those who need to learn to be able to be by themselves or with a warm and sympathetic, calm and understanding human being.

The possession of private property is of great importance to a child. On entering hospital he is likely to feel that he has lost some of his identity. For a child to have his own clothes in his own locker, to be able to help select his own clothes, is extremely important to him.

Coming to terms with oneself is difficult for all of us and we cannot expect children to achieve this perfectly, but the child who is frightened, or who is confused, needs to gain some insight. Some of this will be achieved through treatment, but some of it must be dealt with through the group situation. When a child is able to show his fears and resentments in a group situation it helps him if the trouble can be talked over immediately in a sympathetic way. The nurse should help the child to feel more secure in himself, to learn how to do things with his hands, and to stand on his own feet ; she should work with the child, understand him, and give him respect and love. The greatest healer is laughter and enjoyment, and if the nurse can introduce this into her ward she will be rewarded by seeing the child develop into a mature personality, and a happy and responsible person.

PLAY AND LEISURE TIME

Play is a learning and a healing activity. Through play the child increases his skills, explores, learns to express and develop his own ideas, releases tensions and feelings bound up with his personal relationships, and comes to terms with his experiences.

Destruction of toys will occur and some children will hide them. These the nurse will have to cope with as they occur. Often it is through the child's destructiveness that the nurse is able to assist the disturbed child. If the child is stealing and hiding things away, it is better to know about it in order to deal with it.

Play is a creative activity which develops the imagination ; it is not organized and is developed by the child himself as he plays.

Many children coming into hospital cannot play ; they do not know how to, and the nurse should realize that you cannot teach a child to play, neither can you make him, you can only provide the opportunity and be ready to help, to suggest, and praise, and, if possible, enter imaginatively in his efforts to play.

The problem with a mentally subnormal child is to help him find something he can do and to develop an interest in it. Pencils, paints, drawing materials, games, cardboard boxes, pieces of wood, dressing-up clothes, wooden bricks, and any other oddments which will make useful play material—all these should be available for the child to get himself, so that he does not have to run to a nurse for everything he wants.

Children use play :—

a. *For Pleasure.*—They play because they like doing so, they enjoy all the physical and emotional experiences that play offers.

b. *To express Aggression.*—Children very often work off hate and aggression, and enjoy being able to do so in an environment which does not retaliate. Very often this expression of aggression can be used in activities which have a constructive aim and a social contribution.

c. *To gain Experience.*—Play forms a big part of a child's life. The joys of life are found in play and fantasy, and his personality develops through his play experiences.

d. *To make Social Contact.*—A child at first will play alone or with his mother, other children not being important. Play does, however, provide the opportunity for the initiating of emotional relationships and enables social contacts to develop. Outside of play a child has difficulty making friends, but friends and enemies are made during play.

CHAPTER IX

MOTIVATION THROUGH THERAPEUTIC CARE

INTERPERSONAL RELATIONSHIPS

INTERPERSONAL relationships are two-way processes in which both the patient and the nurse interact as participants, each reacting to a particular situation and observing each other's reaction. These relationships can be broadened to include other patients and nurses.

The expression of feeling between patient and nurse may become therapeutic for the patient if the nurse is skilled in recognizing and understanding why the patient feels, thinks, and acts as he does, and why the nurse reacts towards the patient as she does in each situation. Feelings motivate thinking and behaviour. I am sure most readers will at one time or another have felt anxious in a particular situation and have noticed how difficult it was to communicate adequately with others. This inability to communicate can only be relieved if satisfactory relationships can be established with an individual or a group of individuals.

No one can tell a nurse how to respond to her interpersonal relationships. These aspects of a nurse's response cannot be turned off and on at will. Only general principles and suggestions can be given here, but these added to the nurse's already general knowledge of interpersonal relationships will assist her to deal with most situations.

The nurse should aim at involving all her patients in her relationships. There are patients who are always in the lime-light, usually they make the first approach and there is little danger of them being overlooked. There are, however, large groups of patients who are timid, frightened, and withdrawn, who can easily be overlooked, and who present a challenge to the nurse in establishing relationships.

Failure to establish a relationship with a patient at first should not deter the nurse from making further attempts. One does not necessarily need verbal communication to prove success. The patient's expression will often show the emotionally gratifying experience and this can be highly therapeutic.

Very often just listening to a patient, quietly allowing him to ventilate his feelings, will help to allay his tensions and anxiety. Patients who feel threatened often project this feeling on to others in their environment in order to gain feelings of comfort.

We all have a need to feel accepted by others, and we can accept a behaviour-disturbed patient without approving of his behaviour. It will, however, help the patient to act out his behaviour and how he feels within limits of safety to himself and others. It will be noticed in extreme cases that a patient who breaks a window or destroys his clothing in a fit of temper very quickly settles down afterwards.

It is often difficult for a nurse to accept a patient's obscene language and behaviour, whilst the patient finds pleasure and satisfaction in knowing that his actions are making the nurse uncomfortable. The nurse may represent an authority figure, and perhaps the only way the patient could be accepted in his previous environment, prior to hospitalization, was by conforming and behaving according to the standards of that particular community. In hospital the patient should be free to act out and release his underlying feelings of hostility without fear of punishment. It is helpful for nurses to develop a philosophical outlook regarding a patient's antisocial behaviour and appreciate that he has demonstrated a capacity to respond emotionally.

Behaviour.—All behaviour is meaningful and there is a meaningful explanation for everything a person says and does. If the nurse can understand this it will help her to appreciate the function of helping patients to meet their underlying needs. Meeting a patient's needs is dependent upon her ability to interpret the meaning of an individual patient's behaviour. Any behaviour which reduces or relieves anxiety is rewarding.

Behaviour is never at a standstill owing to the changes which take place causing individuals to react to them. During illness the patient's behaviour changes as he reacts to his environment, treatment, and interpersonal relationships. Understanding of this helps the nurse to be alert as well as to anticipate the patient's response to what is happening.

Some changes may not be difficult for the patient to accept, others require a nurse's support through explanation, reassurance, listening to the patient, and conveying the feeling of trust to him. Some reactions to change are unpredictable owing to the immediacy of the causative stimulus. Changes which can be anticipated offer the possibility of predicting the patient's response as well as of planning a nursing approach. Planned approaches are helpful in reducing or preventing physical and emotional discomfort for the patient.

A change of ward or hospital, even though it is for the better, can have the most devastating emotional effect on a patient, unless he has been adequately prepared for the change so that its reason and advantages for the patient are understood and accepted. Changes in the ward's nursing staff often create anxiety and insecurity, because of his inability to predict the trust of an unknown relationship.

It is important for nurses to be aware of feeling responses to changes in human relationships and to appreciate the importance of establishing rapport in the nurse–patient relationship. It will strengthen feeling of security and alleviate anxiety.

Emotional responses indicate the presence of change, the patient's capacity to adapt, and the need for medical and nursing investigation.

We all need to think well of ourselves. Those people with a feeling of inferiority tend to have their morale and self-confidence undermined at the smallest criticism. Patients need to have their self-confidence and morale boosted from time to time. When they are encouraged they tend to be motivated towards constructive behaviour.

Attention and recognition should be given to the patient upon each contact with the nurse. A busy nurse, too engrossed in her own problems, can inadvertently fail to recognize or speak to a patient in the hospital grounds and have her omission interpreted by a sensitive patient as an act of rejection. One should at all times make the effort to speak and give attention in passing to all patients.

Patients attempt to gain attention and recognition in various ways, for instance, they may refuse to dress, to feed, or wash themselves, or they may feign illness, be meddlesome, distracting, and demanding. Depending upon the particular behaviour expressed, the nurse should respond to the patient's need for attention.

Coaxing, suggestion, paying compliments when deserving of them, joining in games, and anticipating the patient's needs will all help to satisfy the basic needs and help to allay his behaviour outburst.

The need for affection is basic to all human needs. To express liking for another individual it is essential to avoid harsh criticism but instead use tactful suggestion. It is amazing what sincere facial expressions and gestures can do to communicate to the patient that he is liked.

Maintaining consistency, giving reassurance, and setting limitations when necessary all help to give a feeling of security. A patient may react acutely to an absence of consistency in acceptable standards and management. The inconsistency produces feelings of insecurity and the patient is unable to predict what to expect. There should not, therefore, be any conflict between the staff regarding the general approach to the patient.

The patient has a need to communicate with others and to understand other people's method of communication. It is usually necessary for the nurse to adapt her language to the patient's level of understanding.

It is not always easy to understand a patient's conversation; the nurse should therefore listen very carefully to the patient and attempt to identify key words, or syllables, which may serve as clues and help to bring about an understanding of what he is attempting to say.

Observing the patient's gestures, and actions, may also help in understanding his communications.

Talking helps the patient to ventilate his feelings and thoughts, and helps to relieve tension and anxiety.

Listening is an art which may be acquired by those who can learn to restrain the impulse to interrupt the patient's conversation.

Some people have a greater need to be dependent than others; this need may become paramount when the patient finds the problems of living too overwhelming. The longing for dependency, when little is required to obtain life's essentials, often shows itself by a demanding behaviour, inertia, or a somatic illness. When the outstanding need of the patient is to be dependent, the nurse may, within the limits of good judgement, help the patient to meet this need by providing physical nursing care when necessary, and help the patient to make decisions until he is capable of doing so himself.

Many patients have a strong need for independence; these are often people who have lived under authoritarian conditions. The need for independence may be expressed through aggression, negative behaviour, and refusal of nursing attention. Such patients should be encouraged to make decisions and to assume responsibility for self-care.

The nurse's aim must be to induce her patient to acquire habits necessary for social living within his own capacity, and to help him to control his behaviour and not to allow his emotions to govern his actions. The way to teach this is to set a pattern of behaviour for the patient to follow, then those who cannot understand the need for control over their emotions are given new motives which possess the principles of pain and pleasure. These take the form of special privileges and rewards which can either be increased or withdrawn as the need arises. Such negative and positive inducements are constantly needed. The negative inducements are the withdrawal of privileges, with the indirect result that the patient is forced to control his expression of misbehaviour. The positive inducements include rewards and incentives and other satisfying experiences, such as praise and credit given for every good deed and successful achievement.

Through utilizing these two approaches the nurse is cultivating the will in such a way that the desire to behave properly comes spontaneously from the patient, an achievement which the fear of severe punishment would not have.

While trying to inculcate into the patient the need for good behaviour the nurse must not fail to remove any stimuli which will cause the patient to default. For example, boredom, dissatisfaction in the work he is doing, or any lack of affection from the nurse and the group and the resulting security they give, will all be sources of provocation and frustration. Once the provocating factors are removed the incidence of good behaviour will rise.

Happiness is a factor which will induce the patient to resist rebellion and which will crowd out antisocial behaviour.

Important in the contribution towards happiness are : (1) Personal comfort ; (2) Adequate and satisfying diet ; (3) Adequate rest and sleep ; (4) Personal cleanliness ; (5) Comfort and warmth of clothes ; (6) Clean, pleasant, and stimulating environment to live in ; (7) Interesting leisure occupations ; (8) Separation of antagonizing personalities ; (9) Careful selection of all the nursing staff, so that the risk of choosing the wrong types for the work is cut to the minimum.

The selection of nurses is very important and only those with obviously suitable temperaments and habits should be considered, as no one should be allowed to disturb the peacefulness of the patient's environment.

Every member of the hospital staff who comes into close contact with the patients co-operates in moulding the attitudes of these patients into a socially accepted pattern.

Disciplinary policies are so civilized and refined to-day that even certain forms of punishment frequently employed by parents are considered too severe and their use in hospitals is illegal. Beatings are not tolerated, the offenders are dismissed and subject to legal procedure. No patient has his food withheld, nor is he sent to bed without food.

These and similar eliminations restrict the nurse in her efforts to try to maintain discipline, but equally efficient possibilities remain. Any patient found defaulting from the set social pattern in a serious matter is deprived of something held dear, such as freedom and various pleasurable activities.

The forms of rewards and privileges are : (1) Increased liberty within the hospital and city parole ; (2) Seasonal holidays at home or under canvas with the Guides or Scouts; (3) Weekly monetary rewards according to working ability; (4) Facilities for spending their pocket money themselves; (5) Recreational activities; (6) Social activities such as dances and concerts; (7) Excursions.

If the nurse is to give of her best in her work, she must feel secure in her relationships with her colleagues, whether senior or junior, and free to express herself to them. The traditional submission to authority should be replaced by a mutual respect, sharing of ideas, and criticism. The staff should work as a team to ensure the best use of all their gifts and capacities.

Staff ward-meetings should be held under the direction of a group leader, who has experience of group techniques, as often as he or she considers it necessary. Usually one of the experienced medical staff will be qualified to take on this role, a task which will need handling with great care. Without a suitable leader it is better not to hold these meetings; they can be as harmful under the wrong direction as they can be helpful.

At these meetings everyone should be encouraged to say what they feel about the way the ward is being run and the care of the patients. An effort must be made to come to an agreement and, what is important, gain an understanding of what is being done.

At the first introduction of these meetings some frank and uncomfortable things will be said once the confidence of the group has been gained. If the group can accept these with understanding it will produce a better creative staff relationship of mutual respect and kindliness.

Patients should be encouraged to communicate with and express themselves fully to the nurse. Just as the regular staff ward-conferences allow an airing of grievances and provide a place of discussion for their ideas of improvements, the same can be said of a regular patients' ward-conference. These should be held at the doctor's discretion and he should be the leader. All the ward patients who are not too subnormal should be invited to attend. It is obvious that this form of discussion will only be suitable for the subnormal patient and is therefore limited in its scope. It has, however, a great value. There is always a great deal of gossip and discussion amongst the patients about the nursing and medical staff and about the way the hospital is being run. This can be a cause of discontent and result in disturbed and difficult behaviour.

The patients' ward-meetings will bring into the open all the discontent and criticism and will, wherever possible, allow them to be dealt with constructively. The atmosphere must be pleasant and the patients made to feel that they can say what they like and that the staff will understand their difficulties.

It must be expected that the patient will be suspicious and distrustful at first if he has never previously been allowed to air his opinions, and it is important that the nursing staff's attitude should be as receptive as possible, and they should be more ready to listen and understand than to provide answers or pass judgement.

It is important for the nurse to have a high degree of insight, as direct criticism of herself is very likely to happen. She should be willing to face up to the criticism if it is true. Not until she has passed through this difficult phase will a new kind of confidence be established, when the patient will value her as being a real person and not just one put there to maintain control. When such a relationship has been established it will provide better opportunity for the nurse to help and guide each patient, and will result in more stable behaviour.

Through discussion the patient will approve and recommend changes in his daily routine and environment. Because he has had an opportunity to help in organizing his own life he will be a more contented patient. In most wards the patients influence each other, and can build up a feeling of frustration and discontent. The regular ward-meeting provides an outlet for such emotional tension. The atmosphere of the ward cannot fail to benefit from such discussion, and it is inevitable that the nurse and the patient will appreciate the change and respond to it in a pleasant manner.

One of the important channels through which a mentally subnormal patient can express himself is work. If this is interesting, stimulating, and makes use of any particular gift and shows results, it is a great satisfaction no matter how poor the standard of work. So long as the patient can say "This is my own work" that is all that matters. Special care and consideration will be necessary in deciding the ways in which the patient can be occupied. The common domestic tasks, such as shifting ashes, or scrubbing and polishing floors, though essential tasks, can be soul-destroying if they are the only means of occupation, and continue throughout seven days a week without change; they should never become the sole work of any one patient.

There is much hidden talent in many mentally subnormal patients, and when organizing a ward community, individual occupational needs should be ascertained by the nurse. Some patients are better occupied individually, others in groups. Adequate channels must therefore be available for expression of desires and interests. The attitude of the nurse is an important one in her relationship with her patient and his work; only by working with him can she create a helpful relationship. It is always a good plan for her to stop and ask herself the question, "How would I feel and react if I were given this humble task to perform and were watched doing it?" Not to consider the patient's feelings in regard to a certain task, and to give him one against his inclination, can be a frequent cause of resentment, and rightly so. An entirely different relationship will grow up if the nurse works cheerfully and enthusiastically with the patient, no matter what the task. This type of relationship will be stimulating and interesting both to the patients and staff, and will lead to a very happy fellowship, bringing about improved work and contentment.

Patients often use phrases and words without really understanding the meaning and seriousness of them. Obscene language, if once used, will continue to be used by the patient if the nurse is careless in her attitude to this, and allows the flow of obscenity to continue unchecked. Example and correction will quickly eliminate most difficulties; patients look for a lead from the nurse and if that lead is wrong they should not be blamed. Example of the highest order should be given from everyone coming into contact with the patient.

To laugh at the patient and his inabilities is wrong. If he is experiencing difficulties, a helping hand will do more towards building a common understanding in the nurse–patient relationship and a feeling of confidence between them. Persuasion rather than force should be the aim in all approaches to the patient. A tactful but firm approach in some cases and kindly persuasion will, in most instances, overcome aggressive attitudes.

To establish confidence the nurse must use a confident tone, be patient, firm, reasonable in explanation, always consistent, and never lose her temper when discussing the patient's problems with him. Any encouraging facts given to him should be constantly repeated if the need arises. The mind has a great influence over the body—any problem therefore left unsolved may cause varying degrees of physical disability.

The nurse should never criticize the hospital or the medical or nursing staff to the patient. She should take every opportunity of encouraging her patient to have a positive pride in being a member of his ward. An interest in his troubles should be shown. More than likely he will have a self-centred outlook on these. The nurse should point out that others have suffered the same problems and overcome them. A positive approach to overcome them must be shown, otherwise the whole of the nurse's efforts will avail nothing.

If any change in routine has been ordered and the patient is capable of understanding, an explanation as to why it has been changed and how it will affect his life should be given before the change takes place to allow him to begin adjusting himself.

The nurse's relationships with other hospital workers should be cordial. Each member of the hospital's staff, irrespective of how menial his duties, is striving towards the same end, that of rehabilitation of the patient. Good working relationships will help to establish friendships and tolerance of each other, an attitude of mind which will have an indirect benefit upon the patient's life in hospital.

Important Qualities of a Nurse.—

Friendliness.—The relationship between the nurse and patient should be a partnership affair, something that is to be shared. It is the duty of the nurse to find out something about the world of her patient and share in it. Once she has been able to penetrate into the deeper feelings of her patient she will realize how amicable and desperately in need of friendship he is. Friendliness does not call for familiarity; indeed, undue familiarity will destroy the nurse's influence over her patient. Also she should not become emotionally involved.

Dependability.—When a patient has been told that a certain thing will be carried out for him, the pledge should be fulfilled. A promise should never be offered unless it can be made good. When a patient senses dependability in a nurse he feels he has something to grasp that is solid and trustworthy, and will experience confidence and security because of it.

Acceptance of Responsibility.—The nursing care of the patient is the individual nurse's responsibility and she must see that his needs are met, that all necessary precautions to protect him from injury and ill health are taken, and that all prescribed treatments are carried out. If any change in the patient is noted, whether physical or mental, it should immediately be reported.

To see that the doctor prescribes treatment is not enough without seeing that the patient is ready to receive it and does receive it.

Self-discipline.—Whenever groups of people are gathered together there is inevitably noise. The nurse must therefore accept this and be prepared to tolerate it.

Patients will often make accusations about other members of the staff and other patients. The nurse should in all cases reserve her judgement and guard her tongue. She should avoid direct contradiction of the patient's sentiments and try to use reasoning and judgement to practical ends. A nurse who shows her innermost feelings will transfer them to her patient, which will do much to weaken his sense of security. At all costs, personal feelings should be kept hidden from the patient.

The same care and attention should be given to the uncooperative patient as to the well-behaved patient.

Mentally subnormal patients lack the quality of will power and because of this do create more problems. If the nurse recognizes this fact, it will help her to appreciate her patient's behaviour with a greater understanding.

The nurse often has the opportunity to lie to or deceive her patient. A mentally subnormal patient may be very trusting and easily deceived, but once a patient finds out that the nurse has lied to him the very foundation upon which the nurse–patient relationship is built is destroyed, possibly beyond repair.

It is usual for the mentally subnormal patient to have a high opinion of himself and the nurse should not try to repress it. She should, however, encourage the patient to have pride and self-respect. The careless, thoughtless nurse can destroy these two important traits by her tactlessness, and cause distress to the patient.

Argumentative situations between patients and between nurse and patient should be avoided at all costs. The nurse should never allow herself to be drawn into them. To push antagonism only means surrender for the nurse ultimately, but by that time anger, resentment, bitterness, defiance, and a desire for revenge have aroused in the patient assertive and aggressive behaviour.

Observation.—In the nursing of mentally subnormal patients, more than in any other branch of nursing, the nurse's powers of observation are all-important.

Adaptability.—In caring for the mentally subnormal patient, the work provides situations which are completely different from those the nurse usually meets and demand a different form of approach from her. Several different personalities are living together in hospital wards and need to be moulded into a happy group. Only the nurse who is willing to adjust herself to the various needs of her patients will be successful.

Faith in her own ability and a sense of humour will give strength to the nurse when meeting the unexpected and help her to deal with it successfully.

Emotional Maturity.—In emergencies the nurse has often to make snap decisions, yet at the same time avoid acting on impulse.

Not all the help and guidance given by the nurse is appreciated by the patient and only those nurses who are emotionally mature can overcome the disappointments and grief with equanimity.

Cleanliness.—The nurse should aim at providing the patients with standards to live up to, and at creating in the minds of the patients and the public at large the impression of orderliness and cleanliness, to command respect.

Some patients are naturally dirty and untidy and it is only due to the persistent efforts of the nurse that the patient does achieve a high standard of cleanliness in his work and his person. If the nurse setting the example does not follow it herself she cannot complain if the patient ignores her teaching.

Creative Imagination and Enthusiasm.—There comes a time in many walks of life when the recognized formula fails to impress or achieve the goal it was prepared for. This situation can often happen in the care of mentally subnormal patients and calls for a capacity of ingenuity and ability to devise new methods and ideas, even in the face of opposition from patients and colleagues.

For the patient to refuse treatment is serious, but for the nurse to admit failure to administer treatment because of the patient's refusal is more serious, and often indicates that the nurse too freely gives up the challenge.

PLATE VI

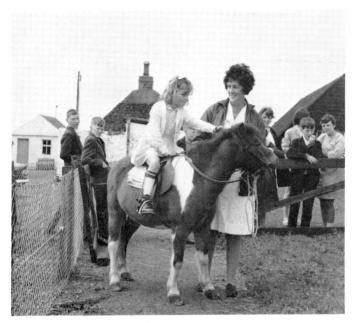

Enjoying the pleasures of her normal sisters.

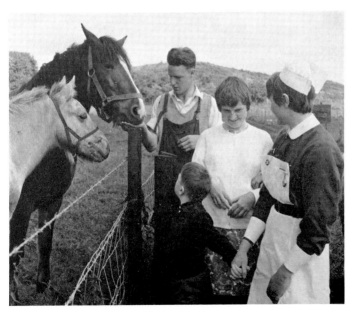

Making friends.

PLATE VII

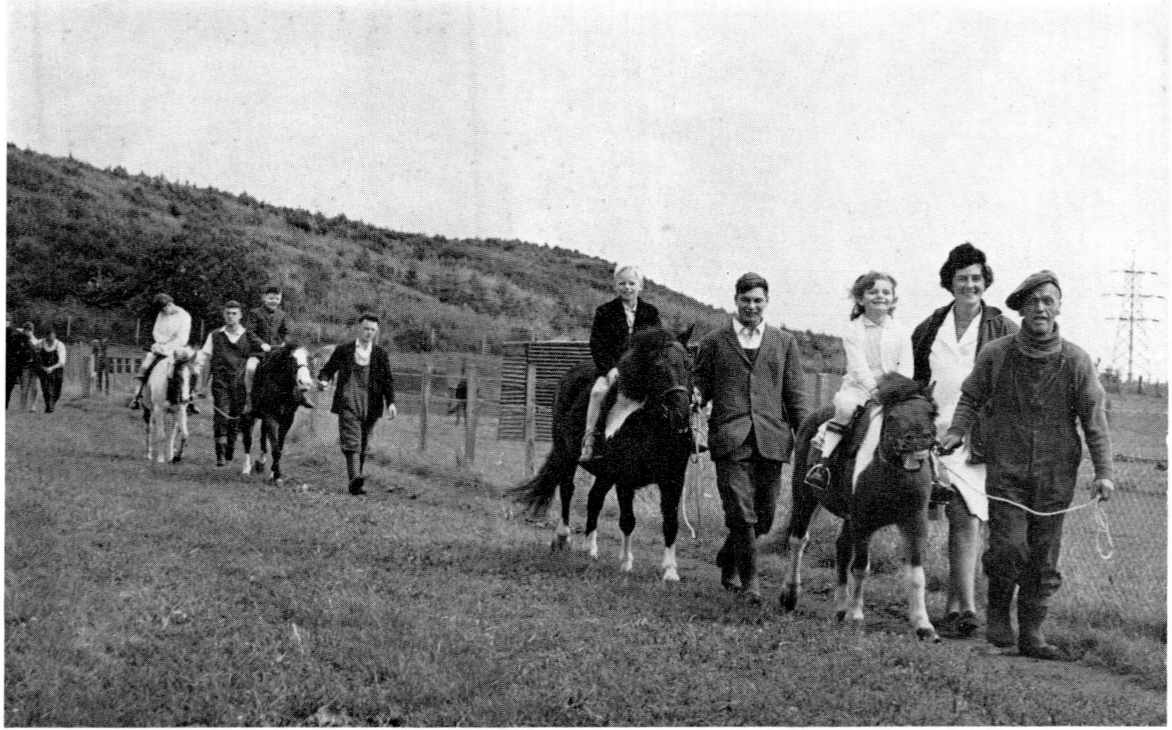

On trek.

CHAPTER X

OCCUPATIONAL THERAPY

OCCUPATIONAL therapy is a basic and most important principle of treatment. Its therapeutic value should be the chief consideration, and all other factors must be secondary and in no way interfere with the primary purpose. The economic side should be taken into consideration only in avoiding unnecessary waste.

Occupational therapy in all its aspects, such as diversional types of occupation and the organized work programme, aims at influencing the patient in his mental state and his habits of work.

Mental State.—The primary effort of the occupational therapy staff and nursing staff is to give the patient a feeling of security. This can often be achieved by providing him with an occupation with which he is familiar, if possible. Friendly relations between himself and the staff are encouraged from the very beginning.

Habits of Work.—Habits of work are taught. The utility departments lend themselves to this desired aim. The patient's capacity for responsibility and co-operation can, in suitable cases, be improved upon. Each patient is taught to take pride in his own work and to value the materials and equipment he uses.

In hospitals caring for mentally subnormal patients there is great scope for occupational therapy. All patients, from the severely subnormal to the subnormal, can derive benefit from suitable and congenial activities.

Many of the severely subnormal suffer from physical disabilities, because of which they have, in the past, been regarded as incapable of enjoying any kind of organized

10

activity.   It is now recognized that excellent work can be done by these patients.

In the majority of cases the patients are young, physically strong, and well suited to various types of domestic and un-skilled work.   It must not be expected that this will be wholly satisfying to the patient.   Some other means of occupation must be available for off-work periods.   This may prove difficult.   First of all, his interest will have to be stimulated and he must be encouraged to express himself in the work he undertakes.   As skill develops he will become more settled and capable of sustained interest.   Nurses will be surprised how many of their patients will, through these efforts, develop a latent artistic sense and desire to create, however simple the form of expression may be.

In addition to being subnormal, the patient may exhibit neurotic or psychotic tendencies, such as mild states of depression.   For this reason training must be by occupation habit rather than by education in its accepted form.   Only by repetition day by day at each stage of the job will he learn. His interest must be maintained so that he does not get bored. This will depend largely upon his relationship with the nurse and the standard of skill he can acquire.   He must be helped to his maximum mental worth, but not forced beyond this capacity.

Use of machines, such as electric floor polishers, vacuum cleaners, etc., can be an invaluable aid, and they will make the unpopular drudgery tasks acceptable and worth while.

If a few appropriate materials are provided, and an incentive offered, the patient will take the lead himself in many instances.

A point often overlooked is that the patients have the physically mature bodies of adults with their accompanying urges and desires, yet because of their mental age and need of care and protection they are deprived of the opportunity to utilize the faculties they possess.

The problem to be met with in subnormal patients is far different from that with the severely subnormal.   Many of the subnormal patients have been unable to conform to the rules laid down by society.   They have difficulty in working peacefully together until they have been taught to understand each other's behaviour.

The hilarious, noisy, and overactive patient will require the very active and energy-absorbing occupations to use up his excessive energies, whilst the depressed type of patient will require a more stimulating occupation which will give the maximum encouragement.

The approach to the patient should be such as to arouse not only his interest but his confidence. There should be an atmosphere of equality in the department where the patient is performing his occupational therapy, and he must be made to feel that his contribution ranks equal in importance with that of the attending staff. Opportunities should be available for a growing interest and an increase in activity to prevent monotony.

Like other forms of treatment, occupational therapy must have medical direction. The medical staff must be in a position to prescribe the correct type of therapy for individual patients and to note their progress, and if necessary be prepared to change the occupation. The occupational therapy department should be under the direction of the senior occupational therapist.

Ward occupations must be organized systematically so as to be suitable for the requirements of patients in bed and patients able to work in the day-room. Where possible a separate room should be available on each ward to be used as an occupational therapy room.

Every member of the ward staff should be aware of the contribution he or she is expected to make to the success of this form of treatment and to attain the desired results.

The occupational therapy staff should co-operate with the medical staff in ensuring that no occupation is prescribed that is obviously beyond the capacity of the patient, or is of a type that does not stimulate interest. If the work allotted is too difficult or has no appeal, then it becomes just another unpleasant task which has to be performed, and fatigue and lack of interest will replace happiness and satisfaction in the job ; the therapeutic effect aimed at will be lost and objectionable traits will make their appearance.

Because of the foregoing dangers it is essential to have a knowledge of the patient's work capacity and interest range and also to have a definite grading of the various occupations and handicrafts.

Ideally, the patient's day should be divided into short periods of different activities, including recreation, sewing, painting, and toy-making, etc. The department housing these activities should be brightly decorated and there should be a background of pleasant music. Environmental factors can cause unhappiness in the patient and may increase any emotional difficulties present, producing deterioration in his performance.

No matter how great or small the patient's achievement is, he will take great pride in it and will develop within himself happiness, contentment, and security.

The approach of the nurse and the occupational therapist must essentially be individual. No matter how backward the patient is, he is an individual person and needs recognition as such. Some patients respond more when carrying out group occupations than when working individually. Others fail to give of their best or maintain an interest unless they are working alone—they lose the sense of accomplishment. The patient possesses something that is 'self' which must be appealed to and satisfied. He must be at first protected from, then prepared to meet, situations that will make demands upon him, and he must be given a healthy outlet for his unavoidable emotional tensions so that he may be able to cope with these.

Occupational therapy can provide an excellent opportunity for developing competence and skills from which will arise confidence, satisfaction, and stability.

It is possible for the patient to have gained some insight into his state, and to react emotionally by unsociable behaviour. A child with normal intelligence has power and opportunity to utilize and further develop his potentialities. A patient who is trying hard but never seems to succeed is upset and becomes unbalanced if accused of laziness, and will retaliate by demonstrating aggressive behaviour ; for example, bed-wetting, temper tantrums, or destructiveness. These will most likely disappear on removing the stress. Encouragement and training directed to better emotional adjustment lead directly to improved behaviour.

In occupational therapy, the standard of work produced should *not* be the criterion. The value is in the patient's sense of positive achievement or even progress.

HANDICRAFTS

The handicrafts section consists of four main units :—
1. Special occupational centres.
2. Ward occupational therapy.
3. The utility departments.
4. Industrial training.

1. Special Occupational Centre.—This is a separate building used solely for the occupational therapy activities. All the advanced and more technical occupations are put into operation here, except the work associated with the various trade-shops, where all the special facilities are available for those tasks, including technical supervision.

The advantages of having special occupational centres are :—

a. It creates a therapeutic atmosphere that might not be achieved in the various wards.

b. It imbues a feeling of specialization in the minds of those patients who have qualified and progressed sufficiently to attend for treatment at this centre.

c. The mere fact of leaving the ward each day to attend a special detached workshop creates an additional therapeutic effect on the minds of the patients.

d. Going to and coming back from the centre creates a normal atmosphere of work for those cases that have progressed sufficiently to become susceptible to the socializing influence of an active environment.

2. Ward Occupational Therapy.—Occupations may be carried out in the ward in the absence of a separate department, or for those patients who require the more intimate and close supervision of the nursing staff.

The crafts used will have to be those which do not require elaborate equipment, are simple and easy to grasp, and non-fatiguing. For the severely subnormal and the excitable destructive patients, rag-teasing is a suitable form of occupation.

The teased material is very useful as engineers' waste and filling for cushions or soft toys. Other ward occupations suitable for the quiet patient are rug-making, knitting, weaving with small hand-looms, basket-making, and other creative work with simple and clean materials.

Bedside Occupations.—These are essential for those patients convalescing from acute illness or for those confined to bed more or less permanently. The range of occupations is limited, but a resourceful and ingenious therapist and nursing staff can further extend the variety ; among those occupations suitable are knitting, crocheting, making soft toys, and soft-leather work. Reading is also an invaluable bedside occupation for those few able to utilize it.

Ward Duties.—These consist of the many daily routine tasks which provide suitable occupation for a number of patients in each ward for the greater part of each day. They are bed-making where the owners of the beds are unable to attend to them themselves, floor washing and polishing, dusting, the transport of dirty and clean linen to and from the laundry and ward, preparation of meals and the cleaning up afterwards, and, where necessary, assisting the nursing staff with low-grade patients and the physically handicapped.

3. Utility Departments.—These consist of the various upkeep and maintenance services of the hospital and are grouped as follows : (*a*) Kitchen ; (*b*) Dining-room ; (*c*) Laundry ; (*d*) Farm, gardens, and grounds ; (*e*) Seamstress's department ; (*f*) Engineer's department ; (*g*) Carpenter's shop ; (*h*) Other specialized departments.

All these constitute a special occupational therapy section and should be under the direction of individuals who are skilled and experienced in the work of their own particular department.

a. Kitchen.—This department will be in the charge of a superintendent cook who will supervise and instruct patients allotted to his charge in the many duties associated with cooking and kitchen craft. The many processes through which food passes from its reception into the kitchen to its destination on the various dining-tables will provide an interesting and skilled type of work which many patients will benefit from. It is work which is suitable for male as well as for female patients.

In the later training of the mentally subnormal patient in preparation for community care the value of the smaller unit for teaching kitchen craft cannot be over-estimated. From this later training the skill of preparing a family meal can be acquired.

b. Dining-room.—The person in charge may be a Home Sister or dining-room supervisor who supervises and instructs the patients in the many duties involved, which include washing and cleaning the table utensils, preparation of tables for the different meals, removal of waste, and the washing and cleaning of the dining-room.

c. Laundry.—There is a great diversity of employment offered and this department will absorb a large percentage of the suitable patients, male and female. The patients sort the laundry and check it into the department, prepare laundry materials, assist with the washing, drying, and ironing, using machines and hand irons. They also prepare laundry for delivery. This department is a good therapeutic aid in its socializing effects.

d. Work on Farm, Gardens, and Grounds.—This work offers an open-air life which varies with the seasons, and can scarcely be equalled by any other section in the amount and diversity of employment offered, some skilled, semi-skilled, and unskilled. Employment includes the working of the different machines in the cultivation of the land, reaping the harvest, care and feeding of the stock, preparing and planting out flower beds, cutting lawns and trimming hedges, and all the multiple activities associated with agriculture and gardening.

e. Seamstress's Department.—This is one of the departments which provides a lasting practical training, whether it be for male or female patients. Most hospitals have a large amount of repair work which is carried out in this department, which also provides most of the bulk of clothing requirements of the hospital. There is a variety of work carried out by machine and hand, all of which suitable patients enjoy doing.

f. Engineer's Department.—This provides only a limited scope for the mentally subnormal patient, but the work has a great attraction for the male patients, some of whom are able to benefit from the training received.

g. Carpenter's Shop.—Many sub-sections can develop from this department, most of which will provide occupations for the mentally subnormal, providing supervision is given. The novelty and variety of the work will stimulate the patient's interest; attention and concentration will be necessary, but because of the interesting nature of the work, there will be little or no mental fatigue.

Serious injuries can be guarded against by restricting the use of certain tools, and providing careful supervision during their use.

h. Other Specialized Departments.—There are other departments such as the bakery, tailor's shop, and the shoemaker's shop, each providing occupational treatment on a small scale, but which do not justify their inclusion here as a separate section.

4. Industrial Training.—The personality make-up of many mentally subnormal patients is complicated by emotional problems which are more incapacitating than their intellectual limitations, while others with lesser intellect are able to achieve more because of their emotional stability and personality assets.

As a rule, the mentally subnormal patient has been conditioned to failure and mistrust from early childhood and is therefore slow to risk himself in relationships. What is often not realized is that he is capable of the same feelings of pride and self-respect as those of average ability. Although he may be very slow in learning, he can master a number of tasks, so long as they are within the limit of his comprehension. Limiting his experience to a step-by-step process will not only facilitate his learning but add the encouragement of multiple successes and mitigate the seriousness of failure.

It is important that all patients who are young enough to benefit from individual training should receive this in separate units which are geared to provide the patient with a realistic programme and a workshop environment which is designed to adjust the personality defects of the individual.

In a well-organized industrial scheme, most grades of patients are able to participate with benefit.

Manufacturers are usually willing to co-operate and will supply tools and materials for carrying out industrial processes in the hospital, though an industrial scheme of this kind will depend upon the kind of industries available. Training should involve a gradual change from simple to more complex work, which at first should be broken down into its constituents. The more varied the tasks learned, the better. One of the greatest problems the nurse will have to deal with will be the patient's dislike of change, the anxiety and sense of insecurity engendered from it. As this is one of the important aspects of industrial life it is imperative that he is taught how to overcome his fear of change. This can be achieved if the patient is kept aware of the aims of the programme and the planned changes he must meet before completion of his rehabilitation.

The success of industrial training and subsequent rehabilitation will depend upon the patient being suitably motivated. Motivation should be stimulated before the patient arrives at the workshop. The nurse should have defined the incentives, both short term and long term, and explained to the patient that at each phase of improvement he will be rewarded by an increase in the incentives he will receive.

The incentives offered must be meaningful and acceptable to the patient. They could include : Payment by results, leading to a personal savings account ; adequate pocket money and the opportunity to spend it as he felt fit ; the right to select and buy his own clothes and other personal possessions ; the right to parole in the community, at least once weekly, but increasing with progress ; holiday leave ; a knowledge of his expected duration in hospital and the prospect of ultimate discharge.

The uncertainty of this latter and of the promises made causes the patient to resist the efforts the hospital is making on his behalf. In this kind of situation, an adequate training programme will very quickly fail.

The following discipline if used when opening an industrial therapy workshop will play an important part in its successful working :—

1. The training should promote successful employment. The work offered to the patient is relevant to industry and the conditions and discipline are the same as those he will meet in any factory.

2. The equipment should be as sophisticated as that found in factories, and the tempo and stresses of work in the unit should be the same as in industry.

3. Local firms should be encouraged to employ the successfully trained patients in their own factories.

4. It is important that the patient is aware of the incentives that are available for good work and work discipline.

5. The selection and training of supervisors and instructors should be carried out very carefully, and no rash selection made.

6. Adequate and regular supervision by social workers is very essential so that any threat of a breakdown can be dealt with before it becomes too serious. The social worker should be keeping the optimal goal of discharge to the community very much to the fore. Progress should be discussed with the patient at least once every week. Points to be defined might include general behaviour, work behaviour, amount of work, quality of work, care of tools and materials, time keeping, and appearance.

Some hospitals have introduced rating scale charts which are kept on display at the place of work, to act as a reminder to the patient for the need to persevere with his work and behaviour.

Many patients fail to adjust in the community due to a lack of understanding of money values. In the past the hospitals have tended to be over-protective and have provided the patient with so little money that he has not been able to gain a realistic understanding of money values. The hospital, having made itself the provider of all things, has removed from the patient's life the opportunity to learn how to plan and organize his life.

A patient with a relatively reasonable discharge potential should be given economic training in a practical situation over a period, during which he will be subjected to the pressures and temptations of everyday living.

CHAPTER XI

REHABILITATION

REHABILITATION is a process of treatment carried out with all patients from the moment of their entry into hospital, and continuing until their discharge into the community, which goal is the purpose of hospital care and after care. The extent to which this purpose is achieved is, however, tempered by the capabilities of individual patients. The pattern of rehabilitation for those able to benefit will be one of several stages of increasing dependency and trust, each suitably graded to produce a stable and reliable patient. Though there is no law for the guidance of those directing the rehabilitation of the patient, the pattern set out below will be the same as that followed in most hospitals for the mentally subnormal.

Daily Employment outside the Hospital.—This is an incentive which motivates most subnormal patients. It has the facility for testing the patient in a loosely supervised work situation and shows up his abilities in a real workshop environment, his relationships with other work people, and his reaction to the community. The placing of a patient in a stimulating normal environment outside the hospital will encourage improvement in most aspects of living. The patient leaves the hospital each day to attend his place of work, and returns in the evening. He receives pay for the work he does, one part of which he is allowed to keep for pocket money, another part goes towards the cost of his upkeep, and the remainder is placed in the bank for him. This he can withdraw when the need arises.

Some patients are a success up to this stage, where they have the controlling influence of the hospital to support them, but are incapable of accepting greater freedom.

Industrial Rehabilitation Centres.—These centres do not officially take the mentally subnormal patient for training. Some do, however, accept in limited numbers those likely to benefit from the training. The mentally subnormal patient is taught some semi-skilled or unskilled work in surroundings which stimulate confidence. The work and the environment, hours of work, and conditions of service are exactly the same as in industry, without the severe competition. Adequate guidance and supervision are given during this training period which lasts from three to four months.

The aim of the rehabilitation unit is to help the patient to adjust himself to a new type of occupation under a more difficult way of living and certainly one he is not used to, as well as to get him accustomed to a new type of discipline which will govern his day in a factory.

The patient may continue to live within the hospital during his training, or he may be resident at home or in lodgings.

Parole.—After a period of controlled behaviour in the hospital, the patient is granted a greater degree of freedom within the hospital grounds, where he is allowed to proceed unescorted from his ward to his place of work, to the recreational hall, the hospital canteen, and elsewhere.

In satisfactory cases, hospital parole will lead to weekly city parole when, in the company of other suitable patients, he is allowed regular visits to the nearest town to do his shopping, visit a cinema or a local football match. In some cases a more generous use of parole is indicated and in these circumstances the patient may be allowed unsupervised parole several evenings each week for therapeutic reasons. A generous use of parole is a practical demonstration of trust and good faith in the patient, and offers the opportunity to test the patient's behaviour in an unsupervised situation. Some hospital authorities prefer that their patients have a holiday at home, where home conditions are suitable, before granting city parole, to test the prolonged reliability of the patient under changed circumstances.

In these cases it is important that a full knowledge of the home and environment is gained before permission for a holiday at home is given. Liaison with the local Mental Health Authority should be sought so that this information may be acquired without raising the hopes of both patient and parents.

Holidays.—After a suitable period of good behaviour by the patient, and where the home conditions are suitable and the parents willing to receive him, a holiday of up to 14 days may be recommended by the Responsible Medical Officer. This is an important stage in the patient's adjustment. It provides him with new experiences in changed surroundings and tests his ability to accept greater freedom.

Long Leave.—All detained patients are eligible for this privilege after a suitable period of controlled behaviour in hospital. The period of this leave is for up to six months, after which the patient must either be returned to the hospital or discharged. Some Responsible Medical Officers use this privilege during the last six months of a patient's order as a test for his suitability for life in the community. The prospect of long leave is a real incentive for good behaviour amongst the subnormal patients, the majority of whom cherish the prospect of living in the community again.

A patient whilst on long leave is under the care of his parents or relatives, the supervisor of his lodgings, or his employer. In all cases the persons accepting him must promise to provide adequate supervision and control while he is in their care, and to notify the authorities if control is being lost or if the patient is failing to adjust himself to his change of environment. His immediate removal can then be made.

Long leave is issued for a period of six months. Whilst the patient is on long leave he is visited regularly by the parent hospital's social worker, or by the Local Mental Health Authority's Mental Health Officer. Informal patients are usually recommended a trial period at home with a promise of readmission should the need arise.

Sheltered Workshops.—These workshops can provide some of the institution's industries and services in which time-tables and contracts have no part, yet the patient being rehabilitated is gainfully employed. The sheltered workshops can also be of great service in providing employment suitable for physically handicapped and epileptic patients. In some hospitals these may be run as group therapeutic and training units, under medical and psychological direction.

New opportunities and challenges are provided for the patient, and his resulting success over them will give him a feeling of social security and a high degree of emotional adjustment.

Occupation Centres.—These centres, under the direction of the Local Health Authority, provide continued training for patients granted long leave by the hospital who are not suitable for industrial occupation. They can continue their training under supervision which will help in maintaining their standard of improvement: attendance is voluntary. Many parents take advantage of the opportunity to be free from the constant worry of their child, and from the mental strain which to some is harmful to health. Transport to and from the centre, lunch, and tea are provided free.

Graded forms of education and all varieties of occupation and entertainment are provided, still aiming at the maximum development of the patient's potentialities and capabilities.

The following difficulties have to be surmounted when endeavouring to place mentally subnormal persons into employment.

Lodgings.—Lodgings are necessary for all patients suitable for life in the community who either have no home to go to, or have homes which cannot provide the necessary stable environment, and it is deemed wiser to board the patient out. Very few people are willing to provide accommodation for mentally subnormal patients.

Wage Regulations and Trade Union Restrictions.—Employers quite naturally select persons who will give a good day's work for a day's pay, and do not require strict supervision. Trade Unions may not look kindly on the small payment scheme for the work done by a mentally subnormal person, and this may require local discussion.

Speeding up of Industrial Processes.—Industry and agriculture are becoming more mechanized and specialized. Bonuses are often given in industry on a team basis, and because the subnormal cannot keep pace, it causes resentment amongst the other team members.

Major changes are taking place in the pay structure of people employed in the hospital industries which are likely to place a greater strain on the employed patient and indeed may inhibit his continued employment in these industries.

Providing that allowances are made for the subnormal and adequate supervision can be given, all the difficulties can be overcome.

RECREATIONAL THERAPY

This form of treatment consists of both physical training and entertainment. Physical training includes gymnastics, callisthenics, and athletics. Recreation includes amusements, games, walks, music, dancing, concerts, reading, and personal hobbies.

It is often difficult to make contact with the severely subnormal patient through the normal channels of persuasion and appeal, but he will respond instinctively through play. This instinctive response is the first step in the socialization of the patient, even though the act is apparently uninfluenced by thought, judgement, or mental effort.

Most stimuli act through the sensations of sight, hearing, and touch, or a combination of these. The majority of patients will respond to visual sensory stimuli and will repeat movements performed in their presence. Those who will not respond may be aroused by auditory and touch stimuli. Through the use of these senses it is usually possible to overcome resistive attitudes.

Recreational therapy promotes and provides new interest which can be graded to suit the needs and ability of the individual patients. Through it dormant interests can be developed. As a result of this development the wards in which these patients live will take on an improved atmosphere. For example, all the patients will be interestingly occupied and their instinctive energies will be sublimated into socially accepted channels. These changes and achievements will inspire the patient's confidence in himself and the care he is receiving, self-trust, and healthy ambitions.

The analysis of the individual activities is as follows.

Gymnastics and Callisthenics.—These activities comprise formal exercises which require to be specially adapted to meet the therapeutic needs of the individual groups of patients.

Gymnastics requires apparatus and special equipment and a high degree of physical fitness of the patients taking part. This form of treatment does not permit much opportunity for grading.

Callisthenics permits a series of graded movements from the very simple repetitive types to the more complicated and difficult types, and is suitable for use with all grades of patients, either individually or in a group. The movements performed should be rhythmical rather than fast and jerky. The use of music facilitates rhythmic movement, providing it is soft so that it does not distract the attention of the operator. It should only indicate the time and rhythm of the movement. Margaret Morris Movement has often been found helpful.

Outdoor Games.—Games as a form of treatment should reach the greatest number of patients possible, as the maximum mental and physical benefits are derived from them. Many patients who will not or cannot take an active part in the various games will enjoy looking on.

The advantage of outdoor games lies in the wide variety of games and sports which can be graded to suit most patients and can be classified into individual or team games.

Athletics.—Special days should be set aside as gala days when the entire hospital population takes an active or passive part in the programme.

The programme should include running, jumping, tug-of-war, relay races, and novelty events, such as egg-and-spoon race, wheel-barrow, and obstacle races. Music can be provided on these occasions by the hospital's orchestra, which may include patients and staff. The realism of the programme will be enhanced if prizes are given to the winners of the different events, and will contribute to the socializing effect of the day.

Indoor Games.—Indoor games form a good substitute for outdoor games, when these are not possible, and there is no

PLATE VIII

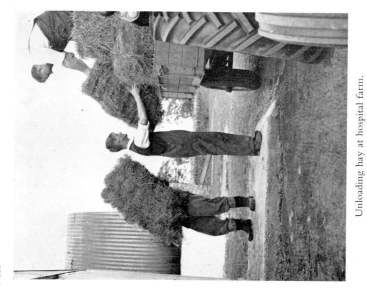

Unloading hay at hospital farm.

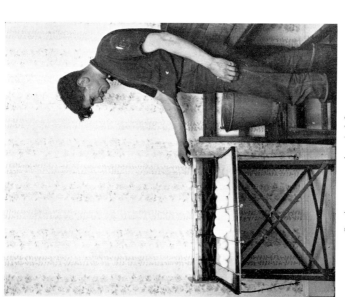

Sorting eggs on hospital farm.

PLATE IX

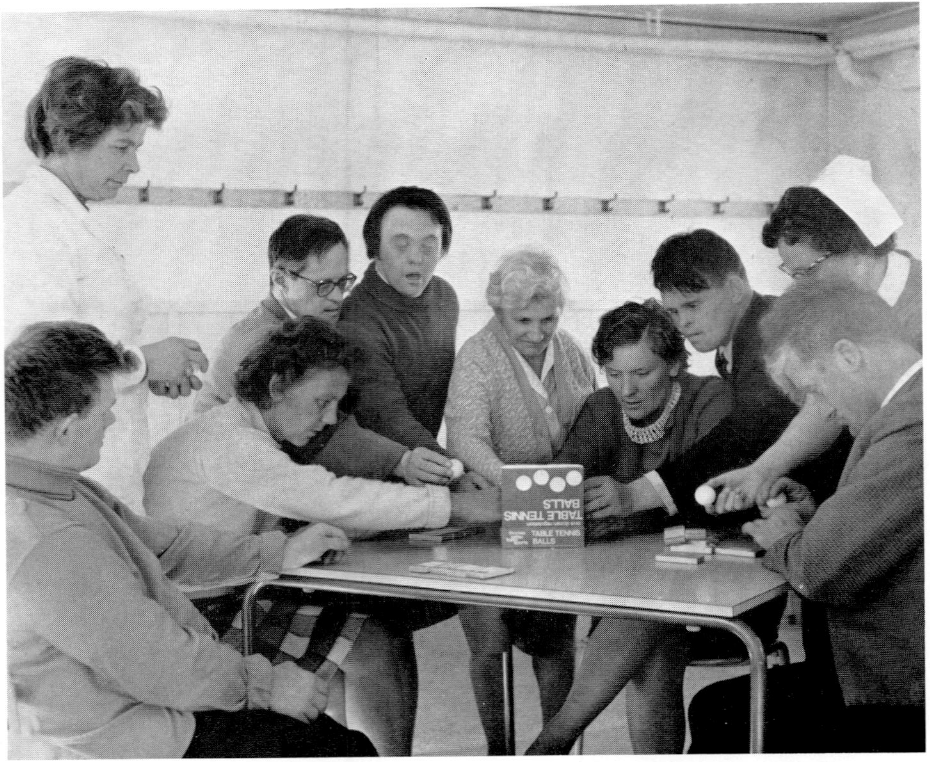

limit to the number and type of game available. The monotony of individual patients playing each other can be overcome by competitors from other wards playing each other.

Musical Entertainment.—Musical forms of entertainment can provide active and passive recreational treatment which can be arranged either indoors or out and can include concerts, wireless programmes, band concerts, choirs, and musical cinema shows. It is through music that the greatest number of patients can be reached. It reacts on their emotions and promotes healthy and desirable moods, and has the advantage of holding their attention where all else fails. It helps to convert an unfavourable atmosphere into one that is cheerful and brighter, and has unlimited powers of entertainment, giving a much needed enjoyment to its performers and listeners.

The active side of music has greater therapeutic possibilities. It creates an outlet for emotional flow and conflict. The performer also develops a sense of emotional satisfaction in his own achievement and a feeling of contribution towards the entertainment of his fellow patients.

Percussion Bands.—Most patients are capable of taking an active part and of deriving great enjoyment out of percussion bands. They also provide enjoyment for all those patients who are only able to listen. Drums, triangles, cymbals, bells, castanets, and tambourines are the instruments used, and the whole orchestra is under the direction of a conductor who is usually a patient.

In the organization of orchestras and choirs the nursing staff can work beside the patients. Their assistance will help to boost the morale of everyone taking part and inspire the patients' self-confidence and co-operation.

Choirs.—Though the number able to take an active part will only be small, large numbers will benefit from the efforts of the few in a passive way. Choirs are mobile and can provide entertainment suited to most tastes. They can travel to the various wards providing entertainment for all those confined to bed. One of their greatest values is being able to lead the singing at all of the Sunday church services, bringing greater joy to all the worshippers.

11

Impromptu Concerts.—At these functions patients are allowed to volunteer to provide musical, vocal, or recitation items. Fixed items should be arranged beforehand to give the concert a start and help the patients to reach a responsive mood. The air of informality should be the high note of the evening.

Cinema Shows and Television.—Suitable films have recreational and often educational value. Television has been found to be of the greatest value as a calming and educational medium.

Dancing.—Dancing is a form of entertainment with a socializing effect that is difficult to overestimate. All grades of patients receive both mental and physical benefits from it. The rhythm of the music stimulates the desire to move with a flowing, swinging action which is aimed at in all muscular activity. This type of movement is the least fatiguing and provides the greatest enjoyment. The types of dancing enjoyed by the patients are ballroom dancing, square dancing, country dancing, and eurhythmics.

Ballroom Dancing.—This can be graded to suit the mental and physical capacities of the patients. It is a form of entertainment which is complete in itself and can be included as a part of the programme of socials and parties. Patients of both sexes can mix under the restraining influence of close supervision and the fear of withdrawal of the privilege for a breach of good conduct. With good supervision the risks involved are slight, and the therapeutic and character-building values are enhanced.

Square Dancing, Country Dancing, and Tap Dancing.—No patients' concert would be complete without at least one of these varieties being used. Mixed or single groups can be used to provide entertainment for the other patients.

Eurhythmics.—Music and actions are combined to provide expression through movement. Memory, muscular movement, co-ordination, and attention are all developed, as well as an increase in knowledge of other parts of the body. The more simple forms can be adapted for use with the severely subnormal patient whilst a more complex form can be used for the subnormal patient.

Walks and Coach Sight-seeing Excursions.—Each of these activities should be a regular feature of the recreational programme.

Walks should be a daily feature when the weather is favourable. The routes chosen should be varied to avoid monotony. Not all patients will be suitable for the active exercise of walking, but those able to benefit from accompanying the walkers in a wheel-chair should be allowed to go. Fatigue should be avoided in those who do take an active part in the walks.

Coach trips should be organized as often as is possible to the seaside, to scenic beauty spots, and to suitable theatre shows. Those patients in a position to do so should be encouraged to assist with the payment of part or the whole of their expenses.

Hobbies.—All patients able to benefit from these should be guided and encouraged in the choice of occupation or interest.

Having a hobby fills up periods of time which would otherwise be used on introspective activities and day-dreaming. Life will become more interesting for the patient if he can be interestingly occupied.

Hobbies commonly met with amongst mentally subnormal persons are the cultivation of individual garden plots—the patient having freedom of choice of cultivation—caring for animals and birds, and stamp collecting.

Ward Activities.—Here the complete co-operation of the nursing staff will be essential as the success of this form of treatment will depend upon their goodwill and support. The nurses should enter into the spirit of the games and regard the therapy as their primary concern. It requires very little skilled experience to get unoccupied patients interested in group or individual games. Bed patients must not be overlooked in the organization ; entertainment must be provided for them as well as for the active patients.

Libraries.—A patients' library can take two forms :—

1. The patient can visit a room set apart where books of all kinds are available for him to make his own choice.

2. The librarian can visit each ward on an appointed day each week with a book trolley filled with books in which the more intelligent patient might be interested.

The types of books most suitable for the mentally subnormal are pictorial books, strip cartoons, simple fiction, and travel and historical books. Books with simple picture illustrations are more suitable for the severely subnormal. The subnormal patient whose command of English is fairly good may benefit from reading the daily papers providing they are suitably selected.

For the very severely subnormal patient highly coloured picture books are most suitable, as these patients have no reading power or understanding of words, but do receive a great deal of pleasure from looking at pictures. Any type of picture seems to appeal to them.

A qualified librarian can be of great benefit to a group of hospitals for the mentally subnormal in that she can organize the library to meet the needs of the patients, and give them advice in their reading. Through her, the resources of the library can be brought to the notice of both patients and staff, and the best supply of books be made available and used to the best advantage.

The nurse's knowledge of her individual patients can also help in the choice of books for them. Through the co-operation of nurses and librarian a successful service can be achieved. Of the two aforementioned library systems, the room set aside for a library is by far the more satisfactory. The patient can help himself and choose from a larger selection of books. It is also introducing the patient into a different environment, where quiet is essential not only for his own benefit but also for that of others.

Hospital libraries can, with co-operation, make a very definite contribution to the lasting rehabilitation of the patient.

SCOUTS AND GUIDES

Special branches of the Scout and Guide movements have been formed to meet the needs of the mentally subnormal patient. Most hospitals appreciate the stabilizing and socializing effect of the two groups and have formed their own Scout and Guide troops.

The aim of the movement is to inculcate an idea of personal service to the community and the acquisition of knowledge to encourage the growth of a sound mind in a sound body. The moral code is practical and is within easy reach of the understanding of the mentally subnormal person, and will act as a guide to behaviour.

It is an advantage if members of the nursing staff can control the hospital troop, because the nurse understands the patient's temperament and knows his capabilities. Through her knowledge she will achieve the best results.

Annual camps are held, when all the members of the troop live under canvas under the direction of the Leader.

Opportunities are available for the Scouts and Guides from the mental subnormality hospitals to enter national competitions. In the handicrafts section the mentally subnormal person usually excels.

One of the greatest advantages to any patient member is that when he leaves the hospital to live outside he may have the opportunity to join a similar organization and the bond of common fellowship will provide him with the friendship and guidance he will need.

PATIENTS' CLUBS

Patients' clubs can play an important part in the rehabilitation of the mentally subnormal and through their influence and discipline most problems can be negatived. The aims of such organizations should be made known to all who are in membership and should include : (1) To inculcate pride in self and a sense of loyalty towards the hospital. Few of the subnormal and psychopathic disordered patients have had reason to be proud or loyal to anything other than themselves. (2) To stimulate a sense of belonging to an organization with some prestige value within the hospital community. (3) To stimulate the patients to think and organize for the future. This faculty is lacking in most patients. (4) To allow the patients a controlled 'say' in the organization of future activities. Many good ideas and a keener interest to take part will result from this participation. (5) A medium through which outside organizations may be invited to take an active part in the hospital's recreational activities in a more intimate manner than is possible in organized field games.

(6) The control of absconding. Patients should be free to attend the club at their convenience and be free to leave at any time up to closing-time. No exceptions should be made to this rule, even for the chronic absconder.

The organization and management of the club should be controlled by a committee of patients, one of whom should be chairman.

It will be necessary for one of the nurses to act as secretary, and she should be prepared to carry out the committee's instructions. A sense of responsibility is inculcated into the greatest majority of patients, even the most antisocial patient, through the club's discipline.

Every member of the committee should be charged with the duty of seeing that the club runs smoothly and in a controlled manner. To attend to the sale of tea, coffee, and biscuits, on club nights; to arrange for outings and the collection of names and fares; to maintain club discipline and to visit any sick members of the club.

A small weekly membership fee should be charged to the members to enhance their appreciation and sense of being a part of an organization.

CHAPTER XII

WARDS AND WARD MANAGEMENT

GREATER efforts are being made to make a more realistic grading and segregation of types of mentally subnormal patients. Specialized wards are being developed where small groups of patients suffering from the same type of subnormality can be given intensive care from a specially selected team of nurses, therapists, psychologists, social workers, and medical staff whose collective efforts make rehabilitation possible for a previously hopeless group of patients, and, at worst, bring about such improvement that the patient can live a more satisfying and happier life than ever appeared possible.

Grading patients according to their nursing needs has the advantages of being able to concentrate nursing effort in wards with the greatest need, offers the opportunity to programme nurse training, protects patients from being exploited by other patients with a higher intellect, and gives the nurse better opportunity to give specialized care.

TYPES OF WARDS

1. **Infirmary Ward.**—It is usual for all the facilities for treating the sick to be concentrated in this ward, where all those who are ill in the hospital are admitted and given the medical and nursing care not possible in other wards. The ward is usually under the care of a qualified sick-nurse who has adequate nursing staff working under her to make possible the high degree of nursing skill necessary.

It should be a rule that once a patient is fit again he is transferred back to his original ward so that his sick-bed is made available and ready to receive the next patient without any delay. Many hospitals prefer to nurse only those patients with minor ailments in their own ward and to transfer those more seriously affected to the local General Hospital, which is more suitably equipped to deal with physical ailments.

2. Sanatorium.—It is not usually a practical proposition for each hospital to run its own sanatorium. Groups of hospitals therefore centralize their tuberculous patients in one hospital of their group where sanatorium treatment is possible under ideal conditions.

It is desirable that a fully qualified sick-nurse be in charge of the sanatorium ward with an adequate nursing staff under her, so that the nurses may avoid the temptation to rush through the work in order to complete it, thereby neglecting to take the necessary preventive measures against infection and thus exposing themselves to unnecessary risks.

3. Children's Ward.—There is movement towards much smaller wards for the care of children and many other specialists such as teachers, speech therapists, and physiotherapists are being invited to contribute towards the total care of the patients. Where this kind of care is being practised the results have proved the changes worth while.

4. Autistic Children's Ward.—Wards of 8–10 patients are being introduced into some hospitals where this type of patient can receive concentrated individual care from the same nursing staff and other specialists over a prolonged period.

5. Severely Subnormal Ward.—Heating in this ward will be necessary on cool summer days as many of these patients are immobile owing to accompanying physical disabilities.

Toilets, wash-bowls, and bathrooms must be conveniently situated and be of such a structure so that they are easy to use, both for the patient and nurse. Constant teaching and supervision are necessary. Any slackness of the routine will be reflected in the patient, whose habits will deteriorate quickly.

6. Ward for Patients with Behaviour Disorders and Aggressive Tendencies.—These wards should have adequate facilities for indoor recreation and hobbies activities, and special rooms set apart for patients who wish to be quiet, to read, or to write letters. These patients should spend most of their time at work or engaged in open-air recreational activities.

7. **Subnormal Ward.**—Patients on this kind of ward often have difficulty in forming stable interpersonal relationships, but with an understanding nurse to guide them and organize their daily lives as far as necessary, they will only require a minimum of supervision. Most of these patients are allowed to leave the hospital to seek their entertainment.

WARD MANAGEMENT

Having been given the delegated authority to manage her ward the Ward Sister must never forget that the product of a hospital is a person who thinks, feels, and reacts. She must meet the pressures, stresses, and anxieties of her job yet retain a calm efficiency and humanity.

It is important to recognize the importance of the valuable principle of delegation and the satisfaction a junior nurse obtains from having individual responsibility for a small group of patients.

The awareness of the principles of management can be fostered by encouraging student nurses to develop qualities of leadership and a critical but constructive approach to the situation they meet.

The importance of team work and corporate effort should become part of the student nurse's thinking, and the concept of management and its application develop as the nurse progresses in maturity and experience.

The nurse should be flexible in her definition of her function since the environment and the individual situation can have considerable effect upon each member of the ward team.

At the beginning of her training the nurse needs to develop her skills in meeting strangers and persuading them to accept whatever nursing attention she has been sent to administer. Her uniform establishes a recognizable relationship with the patient, who usually accepts it as an authority for the order of procedure. The nurse may by instinct or previous experience with a relative at home cajole or bully the patient into acceptance. If she meets with downright refusal she has to decide whether to accept defeat or ask an experienced nurse for aid and may then be told how to deal with the situation.

A successfully managed ward will have all the hallmarks of efficiency :—

1. *Effective in Purpose and Smooth Running.* All unnecessary tasks will be eliminated so that essential jobs will be done well and the maximum of the nurse's time spent with her patient.

2. *Constancy and Regularity.* If the Ward Sister fails to be constant in her approach to staff and patients it will not only cause confusion but the discipline and orderliness of the ward will break down.

Regularity is an essential in the training of the mentally subnormal ; they very often lack any power of reasoning or understanding of what is said or required of them.

3. *Interstaff Relationships and Staff–Patient Relationships.* Respect for each other's individuality and the ability to work harmoniously is essential to any successful enterprise.

4. *Communication.* It is essential that every member of the team knows what the Ward Sister expects of them and to know that in difficulty the Ward Sister will be available to offer advice and help. Suitable means of communication must be made available in order that information may be passed from one to the other without delay or inconvenience in order to avoid it being lost or forgotten.

5. *Delegation of Responsibility.* No Ward Sister is capable of carrying the full responsibility of the ward on her own shoulders and neither is it good for staff morale if she becomes too possessive. She must hand down some of her responsibilities, nothing gives greater satisfaction to a junior nurse than to feel that ' Sister trusts her '. Delegation is also important in the development of team spirit. Any changes in the ward routine will be more acceptable by the nurses if they have had the opportunity to discuss them before their introduction. It is this combined effort which makes the nurse feel part of the ward team.

COMMUNICATION

Entering into some form of effective communication with the mentally subnormal patient is of prime importance in the context of his total care. The nurse cannot claim to understand the patient unless he can communicate with her, nor claim to influence his behaviour unless she can communicate with him. The best method of achieving this is through conversation. This may be difficult at the beginning as his speech may be monosyllabic, he may be completely withdrawn, or he may be deaf and aphasic.

In order to overcome these difficulties, the nurse must endeavour to obtain the patient's respect and confidence; only then will any communication become sincere and meaningful to either person.

If the nurse begins by prying into the patient's most intimate affairs and inmost thoughts she will produce resentment and withdrawal. She is at first a comparative stranger and should confine her conversation to social politeness, presenting herself as a warm-hearted person who is prepared to accept the patient as he is without blame or criticism.

One factor which may dominate the early phase of inter-communication will be the attitude of the patient towards admission to hospital. Nurses tend to forget that, however comfortable and modern their wards are, admission may be an unwelcome necessity and an undesired ordeal to the patient. The anxious may be over-talkative and need constant reassurance; the extrovert may be annoyed at the interruption of his normal way of life and react with hostility, especially if he is admitted compulsorily.

The emotional behaviour of an individual is closely linked with his emotional development. In most mentally sub-normals there is evidence of defective reasoning and invariably there is displacement of emotion. When talking with a patient the nurse must not show obvious emotional reactions to ideas expressed by the patient. This is not to say that she must agree with them or condone his behaviour. She must neither argue with him nor condemn. If he feels resentment from the nurse he will not express himself freely.

Listening is an active process and although it may not make any progress towards resolution of the patient's problems, it will at least give him an opportunity to relieve his tensions and may help him to gain some insight into his own difficulties. Patients may react to their emotional difficulties in many ways, some verbal, others in terms of behaviour; they may show gross emotional disturbance with hostility or complete withdrawal.

The term ' mental mechanisms ' has been applied to the methods we all use to attain mental harmony. Examples of these are rationalization and projection, which permit the individual to endure his plight or make adjustment to his difficulties so that life can continue, self-respect can be maintained, and a feeling of security, however precarious, can be achieved. Many people may as the result of early environment, mistrust others, belittle themselves, and feel inadequate to deal with the stresses of their life. They lack self-confidence and find difficulty in expressing themselves. If the nurse is asked to comment on the conversation of the patient, allowance must be made for this and an objective assessment made. It is easy to colour a report by one's own prejudices and preconceived ideas. If a nurse's vocabulary, particularly of technical terms, is faulty or inadequate, she is not able to carry out her work fully. Sometimes a patient may ask the nurse for advice ; if it is within her province and the nurse is aware of her own limitations of knowledge and experience, it may be given, but wherever there is doubt the nurse must seek the advice of someone with more experience or more authority.

Ward meetings give an excellent opportunity for the pooling of experience and for the patient to express his wishes and to seek guidance. They also enable the nurse to gain insight into her own attitudes, and her place in the ward team. In order to get the best out of them the nurse must learn to take an active part and to contribute. Unless the nurse can express herself verbally and in writing in such a way that her thoughts are well put over, her meaning clear, and her use of language accurate, neither her conversation nor her written reports will have much significance.

The essential function of the nurse in a mentally subnormal hospital is to appreciate the patient as a person with his own basic personality, social and family background, and intelligence on which is superimposed mental subnormality, to make contact with that patient, and to understand him. This can only be done if communication is good. Efficient communication between persons is not easy and it is made more difficult by mental subnormality. The nurse must therefore become an expert in this special field and practise constantly the art of communication. Some of the present-day problems within hospitals for mentally subnormal patients can only be solved by the members of the staff themselves.

Nurses should be able to identify themselves with their patients without becoming emotionally involved. This is not easy, but is so essential if the best results are to be expected. It will require a great deal of experience for a new student nurse to develop this art. Often the first inclination of all new staff is to treat the subnormal patient as if he were a pet dog, with a real affection but without a true human relationship. The demands placed upon all nurses are great, but should not be insurmountable, and with increasing experience the nurse will gain confidence in herself and be able to lose herself in her patient.

The Ward Sisters and Charge Nurses are key figures of hospital life. It is around them that the daily lives of the patients revolve ; it is they who organize the daily routine, who lay the foundation for the daily care ; but it is the task of all the ward staff, including the junior student nurse, to build upon that firm foundation. It is a good plan for a policy to be prepared by the Ward Sister in consultation with her staff, so that it becomes a combined effort and results in a greater all-round co-operation. A nurse should always have confidence in her senior staff, and always feel that she can go to them for advice and assistance at any time, and feel confident that her call for help will be answered in a practical way.

Much is being done for the mentally subnormal patient and much more can still be done by those willing to devote themselves to the urgent needs of their patients.

The Management of Behaviour.—Instructions to the mentally subnormal patient should always be positive. Persuasion, encouragement, and rewards have greater value in inducing the patient to work than punishment has. Work performed because of the rewards it will bring will be far better done, and carried out with greater joy and ease, than will work done under the fear of punishment.

Commending the patient for good behaviour will be more effective than scolding him for misbehaviour. Through using persuasion, encouragement, and rewards the nurse is emphasizing and spotlighting goodness and helping the patient to focus his attention on correct behaviour. If the nurse can disregard misbehaviour, yet at the same time approve of good behaviour, the patient will behave better. A patient should know what is expected of him and the requirements should be consistent; rules of to-day should hold good to-morrow. If the nurse is constantly changing her mind the patient will not respond as required because his mind can only grasp consistency.

It is important that the nurse avoid issues with her patients. If she does not she will only forfeit the respect of the remainder of them. Waiting until a stubborn patient has calmed down before discussing his problem with him avoids issues and is more effective.

Threats, when made, are rarely carried out, and the patient is quick to realize this, which encourages him to continue in his waywardness.

The nurse will often meet the shy, withdrawn patient, a condition resulting from continued failure in school-work, social contacts, and occupational interest. To overcome this shyness the nurse must provide a stimulating environment and give the patient interesting occupations in which he can have a sense of achievement, and in which he can share with his fellow patients. Opportunities for successful friendships will thus be offered.

These factors will help the patient to react more normally to his environment and to the other patients and nurses.

The Management of Aggressive Patients.—It is important that the nurse does not take offence at what the patient says to her, no matter how serious the remark. The sole reason for a patient making provocative remarks may have been to arouse the nurse to aggressive behaviour, and by so doing attract attention to himself and gain an expression of sympathy or admiration from the other patients.

A violent patient will often give up a struggle when two nurses are present, and if a struggle does ensue the more nurses there are to handle the situation, the less likely is the patient to be injured. If assistance is not immediately available it is the nurse's duty to call for help. By doing so she will not be showing any signs of weakness, but showing common sense and a true understanding of her patient.

Any struggle should be reported immediately to the Ward Sister so that any injuries that may have resulted may be discovered and treated.

Under no condition should the nurse retaliate. Ill-treatment and neglect towards mentally subnormals is a punishable offence under the Mental Health Act of 1959.

Nurses should never be left single-handed with troublesome or violent patients, so that any possible aggressive outbursts can be managed, in most cases, from the realization that there are sufficient staff to keep control. It does sometimes happen, however, that a patient makes an aggressive or homicidal onslaught on another patient or on the nurse when help is not available. Such an incident is fortunately rare; however, the nurse should know how to handle the situation if it should arise. The nurse who keeps calm and does not panic under such conditions is the one most likely to handle the patient successfully and with the least disturbance.

Where possible, an attempt to talk the patient out of his intentions should be made, but where this fails and the patient makes an attack, physical restraint will have to be used only in such a way as not to be painful or likely to injure the patient. An attempt to call assistance must be made.

Once the patient has been restrained he should be put to bed so that he can calm down in quiet surroundings. The doctor must be informed and will give necessary instructions after seeing the patient.

Care of the Keys.—Anything kept under lock and key must be considered to be private or confidential, or to be drugs or equipment which in the wrong hands would be dangerous. To prevent misplacement of the keys, the nurse should have them attached to her person in such a manner that they can be used with ease but be impossible to leave behind. Any loss of keys must be notified to the Matron immediately. Patients should not be allowed to handle the keys.

Bathing.—When the nurse is detailed for bathing duties, she should first of all read the rules of bathing which are usually to be found hanging in the bathroom, to make sure that she is fully conversant with them. These rules are simple and if adhered to accidents will be prevented. They are as follows:

1. Run cold water into the bath first and add hot water to the desired temperature of 90°–98° F. (32°–36° C.).

2. Never add hot water while the patient is in the bath.

3. Do not allow any patient to have possession of the hot-water tap key. This key should be removed and locked away after use.

4. Do not leave the patient alone in the bathroom whilst there is water in the bath.

5. The depth of the water should only be sufficient to cover the patient's thighs.

6. Whenever possible, two members of the nursing staff should be in attendance when epileptic and physically handicapped patients are being bathed.

7. If a patient has an epileptic fit or collapses during his bath, the nurse must :—

a. Keep the patient's head above the water.

b. Remove the plug.

c. Call for assistance and notify the doctor immediately.

d. Dry the patient.

e. Wrap the patient up warmly.

f. Remove the patient from the bath and put him to bed.

Unless there are medical instructions to the contrary, each patient should have at least one bath each week. There are those who will require daily baths to protect their skin against irritating excretory substances and to prevent unpleasant odours. Shower baths can be of great value especially when nursing the incontinent patients.

Night Duty.—It is usual and necessary for the student nurse to spend some of her training period on night duty, which provides her with a great opportunity for improving her knowledge of patients.

Night-time to most people is a time when it is easy to discuss problems, hopes, and fears with other people. The mentally subnormal patient will welcome a nurse who is willing to give the time and a sympathetic hearing to him. Bonds of friendship can thus be bound even more securely—an attitude that should be encouraged. One is aware that staff shortages may make it extremely difficult for the nurse to devote as much time to each patient as she would like.

A great deal of knowledge can be gained about a patient during the hours immediately before sleep. Any discussion of confidences should be treated seriously and not be divulged to anyone other than the Ward Sister and the Medical Officer.

The night nurse on arriving at the ward should first of all read the Day Sister's report, question the Sister on any matters that do not appear to be clear, then visit each patient in the company of the Sister to satisfy herself that the patient, windows, doors, and equipment are as reported. This does not mean that the nurse is questioning authority, but that the patient's welfare is being safeguarded.

Duties performed by the nurse during the night should be carried out as quietly as possible so that the patients are not disturbed. Rubber-heeled footwear should be worn and any offending squeak of the leather treated so as to avoid undue noise.

The habit-training of incontinent patients must continue during the night as well as the day, and all reasonable care must be taken to protect the patient against catching cold. Slippers and dressing-gown should be worn during these visits to the toilet and all rules of personal decency should be adhered to.

Epileptic patients and patients known to be restless and possibly aggressive should have their beds near the night nurse's desk; the nurse is then on the spot if anything untoward happens.

Restless patients should be encouraged into sleep rather than have to rely upon sedative drugs. Often all that the patient needs is peace of mind and assurance from the nurse. Failing this a warm drink will often produce a feeling of drowsiness and a desire to sleep. All irritating noises should be eliminated as far as possible. Ventilation of the dormitories should be adjusted as required to prevent overheating and a stuffy atmosphere. Precautions against draughts should be taken.

12

The night nurse's report must be in writing and be made on each patient. As emergencies arise and are dealt with a full and detailed account should be made immediately so that the risk of forgetting important details does not arise.

Daily Routine.—To avoid waste of time, most Ward Sisters have a detailed time-table to suit all who work in the ward and to suit the requirements of the patients. A well-planned routine and a strong sense of timing in a nurse will accentuate the rhythmical working of a ward.

As soon as the Ward Sister has received the night nurse's report she assembles her staff and reports to them on her patients, and gives them instructions concerning any special nursing treatments and any special routine ward duties she wishes to be carried out.

Care of the Dormitory.—All the beds are made, the patients being encouraged to do this themselves if capable. The bed-patients are washed or bathed and their beds made, and they themselves left comfortable. When this is completed, the dormitory is swept, cleaned, and dusted by those patients who are not detailed to prepare the dining-tables.

Care of the Day Room and Annexes.—After breakfast, all the patients, with the exception of a few suited only to work in their ward, go to work in the various workshops of the hospital. Some may go to work outside the hospital grounds.

Under the nurse's supervision, and with her help, the remaining working patients will perform the various domestic tasks.

Adequate cleaning materials and equipment should be available to avoid the temptation of using wrong items of the ward stock for cleaning.

The nurse must see that the washing-up after meals is carried out properly.

The shelves and floors of the kitchen and larder should be washed daily and any excess food disposed of.

Day rooms and annexes should be well ventilated to prevent stuffiness, unpleasant odours, and the risk of infection.

Flowers in the ward should be rearranged and freshly watered daily.

If the nurse tidies up as she goes along and uses common and artistic sense, the ward will always look tidy and the tasks of keeping it clean and pleasant will be made easier and result in an improved effect upon the morale of the nurse and her patients.

Soiled Laundry.—This should be sent to the laundry daily in its appropriate containers and be marked ' soiled laundry '. To avoid the shortage of ward-linen it is usual to collect the equivalent amount of clean linen from the laundry or ' linen exchange department '.

Ordering Daily Stores and Special Diets.—Such things as tea, sugar, milk, butter, special diets, and new drugs prescribed by the doctor are usually ordered daily. Topping-up services are now being introduced into hospitals which eliminates a considerable amount of bookwork and hoarding. Greater use and economies of equipment, material, and staff have been made where these services have been made available.

Medicines.—It is a safeguard that if a nurse has not passed her preliminary examination she should not be allowed to administer medicines alone. The nurse should know the liquid measures and their comparative values and understand the meaning of the prescription and abbreviations, both on the ward medicine chart and on the medicine bottle.

Immediately a patient is ordered a drug it is the nurse's duty to acquaint herself with all that is known about its action and potentialities. She must know :—

1. The prescribed dose, and the maximal dose that can be given.

2. The method of administration and any special points arising from it.

3. The expected effects of the drug.

4. The side-effects which can occur.

5. The possible ill effects it may produce.

The nurse is responsible for the safe keeping and storage of all drugs. When administering a drug to a mentally sub-normal patient she should remember that identification of the patient will not be easy in every case and that every effort must be made to clarify a patient's identity and the drug he has been prescribed.

Most hospitals have their own rules governing the times for giving medicines. Great care must be exercised to ensure that they are given at the times and in the dosage stated on the prescription chart, and to the correct patient.

Patients' Letters.—

Section 36.—No restrictions are normally placed on the receipt by patients of letters, although under this Section the Responsible Medical Officer has authority to withhold from a patient detained in hospital any postal packet addressed to him if the receipt of the packet would be calculated to interfere with his treatment. Any postal packet withheld must be returned to the sender.

Authority is given to the Responsible Medical Officer to withhold from the Post Office any postal packet addressed by the patient : (*a*) If the addressee has given notice in writing to the Managers of the hospital, or to the Responsible Medical Officer, requesting that communications addressed to him should be withheld, or (*b*) If it appears to that Officer that the packet would be unreasonably offensive to the addressee or is defamatory of other persons (other than persons on the staff of the hospital), or would be likely to prejudice the interests of the patient.

Every patient has the right to have any letter sent unopened to any of the following :—

1. The Minister of Health.

2. Any member of the House of Commons.

3. The Master or Deputy Master or any other Officer of the Court of Protection.

4. To the Managers of the hospital.

5. Any other authority or person having power to discharge the patient.

6. A Mental Health Review Tribunal, at any time when the patient is entitled to make application to the Tribunal.

7. To any other class of person the Minister may prescribe by regulations. The provision of this Act applies to the informal patient and to patients subject to guardianship.

Fire Precautions.—The thought of a fire strikes terror in the hearts of many people, as so much devastation and loss of life occur in a very short space of time. Adequate fire-prevention measures and fire-fighting procedures should be carried out unstintingly.

Fire Prevention.—

1. All electrical equipment should be periodically inspected to test its efficiency and to correct any flaws. However, any defect noted during daily work should be reported to the engineer's department and the fire officer. The insulation around electric wiring does not last for ever, and though we may be getting good service we may be lulled into a false sense of security. It should be a rule that only an electrician should add extra wiring and plugs to already existing circuits and repair fuses. Proper earthing of electrical equipment is essential.

2. Proper maintenance of all types of equipment, especially those worked by gas and electricity.

3. Suitable storage for all combustible materials, such as floor polish, cleaning fluids, paint, paraffin, and waste paper. Metal cupboards will be more suitable and safer than the usual wooden ones.

4. Frequent cleaning and inspection of all linen cupboards, attics, basements, and storage cupboards to see that they are being properly used, and that no unauthorized storing takes place.

5. Periodic fire-fighting practice within the hospital so that the Fire Brigade may become familiar with the hospital, the types of ward, and the equipment and its location.

6. Preparedness for an emergency by regular fire drill, both for patients and all the hospital staff. Instructions dealing with each member on each ward must be set out so that no confusion occurs when the need arises.

7. Most psychiatric hospitals are having to cater for a greater number of patients than was originally intended, which in itself is an added risk and requires its own system of dealing with emergencies. All possible exits must be kept clear and procedures for the handling of greater numbers of patients must be practised.

8. Oxygen is used in most hospitals. In the wards or departments where it is being used the following rules should be strictly adhered to :—

a. Smoking or naked lights should not be allowed.

b. Electrical equipment, because of the possibility of sparking, may be banned.

c. Metal trolleys should be earthed by a piece of metal chain trailing on the floor.

d. Oil should never be used on the equipment.

e. Inflammable material should not be in close proximity.

9. All fire-fighting equipment should be checked at least twice every year.

10. A fool-proof method of notification of an outbreak of fire, speed of notification, and response to the fire-alarm are essential precautions and may render a fire harmless.

Careful Use of Fire-guards.—All ward fires, whether coal, gas, or electric, are a potential danger and must be treated as such. Every fire in use must be shielded by a securely attached guard which must be kept locked. At times when the fire needs attention the nurse must first gather together all her requirements for the job before unlocking and removing the guard, and before leaving the fire she must replace the guard and lock it in position. Attending to fires on the wards should be the responsibility of the nurse.

Preparing and Lighting Fires.—In preparing fires only the orthodox materials such as paper, wood, and coal should be used. Slightly inflammable materials, apart from being expensive and wasteful, are dangerous.

Transferring burning coals from one fire-place to another should never be allowed. There is a great danger that some of the burning coals will fall off the shovel and set alight some of the furnishings. The nurse will be incapable of dealing with this situation because of still having burning coals on her shovel.

Safety matches should be used by the nurse because of their difficulty in lighting from ordinary friction.

Fires should not be built up too high and should only be lit in rooms that are being used. A burning, neglected fire can be a veritable danger.

Fire-fighting Procedures.—In the event of a fire occurring, the following routine should be observed in that section of the building affected :—

1. Give the alarm.
2. Remove all patients from immediate danger.
3. Close all doors and windows to prevent the spread. This applies also to the exits, though they must not be locked.
4. All available staff not required to attend to the patients should use the fire-fighting equipment in an attempt to localize the outbreak until extra help is available.
5. Avoid panic. This can cause more danger to the patients than the actual fire.

CHAPTER XIII

NURSING ASSIGNMENT

CASE ASSIGNMENT

DURING the course of her training the student nurse will be detailed to carry out ' case assignments '. This will involve a more detailed study of individual patients with the permission of and in consultation with the ward sister and Responsible Medical Officer. It is a useful exercise for all nurses to undertake voluntarily failing the direction. The end-result should be a more detailed intimate knowledge of various types of patients and, developing out of this, a closer relationship between the nurse and the patient.

The following sequence of inquiry will be helpful in avoiding omissions of vital importance :—

1. Social History.—This will be obtained from the official records and will give a comprehensive report of the social worker's interview with the relatives, recording the family history, the child's developmental history, home environment, parent–child relationships, and factors leading to the need for hospitalization.

2. Detailed Observation of the Patient.—A detailed description of the living habits of the patient should be included here. Mention should be made of the patient's toilet habits, eating habits, degree of self-care, work habits, relationships with staff and patients, and response to discipline and hospital routine. What are his hobbies and interests, and what peculiarities, if any, does the patient possess? Careful note should be made of the patient's response to medication, describing carefully and accurately any abnormal reactions noted.

3. Behaviour Problems.—Very often the nurse will be able to isolate the irritating factor causing the outburst and from her close observation she may be able to suggest possible solutions.

The nurse's report on her case assignment offers useful material to discuss at a case conference, where the psychiatrist, as the group leader in the therapeutic team, will, with the co-operation of the team, be able to formulate effective and progressive care for the particular patient.

NURSE'S NOTES

The nurse's notes, written clearly and accurately, recording her observations of her patients, have extreme value to the doctor when assessing the patient's future treatment requirements.

During the nurse's daily contact and observation of her patients valuable information concerning the patients' present mental and physical condition can come to light and can all too easily be lost and forgotten unless the nurse is prepared to include the keeping of notes as part of her daily task.

As a guide to note-keeping the nurse may find the following advice helpful and it may give her something upon which to form a basis for her observations :—

1. To give daily information about the patient's behaviour.

2. To give information concerning his relationships with other patients and staff.

3. To indicate his working ability and degree of self-care.

4. To record any unusual characteristics or physical signs.

5. To give detailed advice on the patient's feeding habits and bowel action.

6. To record anything that appears to be unusual.

7. To record reaction to medicine.

8. To record observations which will form a basis for her own research when case files are available to her.

When a nurse has been diligent in recording her observations she is justified in expecting them to be used ; if not, she will very quickly lose interest and cease to compile notes in the future. The notes made should be brief and to the point, but capable of conveying accurately the meaning intended. The use of simple English language is preferred to technical terms, and concrete facts are always of use, whereas generalizations have very little value. It is always helpful to the doctor to have quoted the exact conversation held with the patient who appears to be suffering from anxiety, delusions, or hallucinations.

All notes should be signed and dated by the nurse who has prepared them; then, should the doctor wish for further information concerning the report, he will know whom to consult.

SOME FEEDING DIFFICULTIES

Vomiting.—There are patients who vomit readily and there are those in whom the vomiting becomes an established habit without any underlying pathological cause. It can, of course, have a psychological cause, as in cases of rejection. Many severely subnormal patients put their hands in the mouth to produce vomiting. This they may do to relieve the discomfort of food residue in diverticuli of the œsophagus or in hiatus hernia. The possible reason should, however, be investigated and often the observant nurse will be able to find it. A wide range of causes may include the gulping of food too quickly, frustration, finger-sucking, unsuitable food, and air-swallowing. Some patients may have what is described as a ' slow-emptying stomach '.

Regurgitating.—This should not be confused with vomiting. In these cases the patient returns a small amount of feed as he brings up wind or between feeds. It is rarely of importance, but it is often a sign that he is eating a little too much.

Ruminating.—This is a condition which is difficult to control. The patient is usually over-active and appears to enjoy the taste of the regurgitated food, which he brings up in mouthfuls and which he moves around in his mouth as if 'chewing the cud ', finally depositing it on the floor. This habit can be very persistent and considerable amounts of nourishment can be lost. Unless care is taken these patients very quickly become dehydrated.

ELIMINATION

Many subnormal people suffer from a deficiency of muscle tone, and because of this they do not sense the signal for bowel evacuation; they therefore fail to attend to this important function and sometimes the delay continues until an impaction of fæcal material occurs. A distended abdomen due to impacted fæces is often mistaken for a surgical emergency or ascites.

Lack of ability to chew in some patients causes them to take less ' bulk ' in the diet, bulk being that part of the food eaten which is indigestible and which passes through the intestinal tract, causing a formed stool.

Proper bowel evacuation is important, and many patients require constant observation and encouragement in an effort to avoid chronic constipation becoming established. The avoidance of constipation can be aided in several ways :—

1. Exercise.—The mild exercise necessary for walking assists in the mechanical passing of food through the intestines. A swimming pool offers a means of exercise, even for patients who cannot walk. A patient does not have to be able to swim to exercise in the pool ; by holding on to a handbar or being supported by a nurse he may move his whole body with the least effort. The pool should be heated and proper precautions should be provided for the patients' safety. No patient should be allowed to stay in bed unless physical illness indicates otherwise.

Floor mattresses should be laid out, the patients suitably dressed and encouraged to move freely on the mattress without being impeded by bedclothes. Passive movements carried out by the nurse can be of valuable assistance.

2. Fluid Intake.—The nurse should see that all her patients take sufficient fluid with their meals and between meals. Without adequate supervision it is easy for patients in large wards to become dehydrated. Drinking the water from wash basins, fire buckets, toilets, and from the bath may mean that the patient is just plain thirsty ; it has no psychological significance.

3. Fresh Fruit.—Fresh fruit, though often the cause of loose stools, should never be denied the patients, as, apart from containing a high bulk content, it also is the main supply of vitamin C which is essential for health.

4. The Addition of Bulk to the Diet.—Foods which provide bulk in the diet are : whole-grain cereals, leaf vegetables, fruit pulp, and any other foods containing fibres. Thoroughly cooking and chopping makes the use of these foods possible in the diet of patients with chewing difficulties. Finely shredded cabbage may be used in salads. Whole cereals when cooked need little chewing.

5. **Natural Laxatives.**—Fruit juices, especially prune juice and fig juice, have a laxative effect. The doctor may recommend that these be added to the diet or given in small amounts before breakfast. Individual tolerance to laxative juices varies. Too large an amount produces diarrhœa and intestinal pain.

6. **Enemas.**—Continued use of enemas may interfere with normal bowel movement, cause gradual dilatation of the colon, and wash out desirable mucus which is the natural lubricant of the colon. However, some mentally subnormal patients may need help from enemas.

If the doctor orders enemas, he will order the kind and amount. Commercial disposable preparations are now on the market. These premeasured enemas have complete directions printed on the package and may be given at room temperature.

7. **Habits.**—Regularity in elimination is important. Establishing regular times for evacuation is part of bowel training. The high-grade as well as the low-grade may need reminding. The doctor may order suppositories at designated times to assist the formation of regular habits.

SUBSTANCES EXCRETED BY THE KIDNEYS IN METABOLIC DISEASES ASSOCIATED WITH MENTAL SUBNORMALITY

Doctors are increasingly requesting the nursing staff to collect 24-hour specimens of urine to assist them in their research into the causes of mental subnormality. In several metabolic diseases known to be associated with mental subnormality characteristic substances are excreted in the urine, and it is often the finding of an abnormal metabolite which furnishes the first clue to the aetiology of such disorders.

The abnormal metabolites found in the urine of mentally subnormal patients with metabolic diseases include : phenylpyruvic acid ; phenylalanine ; orthohydroxy phenylacetic acid ; galactose ; amino-acids (increased amounts) ; tyrosine in large amounts ; chondroitin sulphate ; leucine ; isoleucine ; valine ; proline.

INVESTIGATION OF URINE

The examination of urine is one of the oldest as well as one of the most constant of aids to diagnosis, yet only of recent years has it been of assistance in the diagnosis of mental subnormality. Practically every deviation from normal is quite clearly understood. The methods of examination include inspection, combined with physical, chemical, and bacteriological tests. These tests provide the most general means of estimating the efficiency or otherwise of kidney function and the chemical excretion of the body.

The collection of specimens and simple routine tests are part of the nurse's routine duty ; special examinations are carried out by the pathologist.

Collecting Specimens of Urine.—A specimen is obtained and tested soon after admission in every case and at specified intervals thereafter.

A single specimen is regarded as being the urine passed at one voiding. Usually only about 5 fluid ounces (about 145 ml.) are put up for examination, and this, in males, may be a mid-stream specimen. The amount to be tested is put into a clean specimen bottle which is labelled with the name of the patient and the date and time of its collection. The name of the hospital and of the ward must be added if the specimen is to be tested in a laboratory which is not for the exclusive use of that particular hospital.

If the examination is for its bacterial content, it is important that the glans penis and the urethral meatus be cleansed with sterile distilled water, and that a mid-stream specimen be collected in a sterile flask, the first urine to be voided having washed out the urethra. The flask is then plugged with cotton-wool that has been passed through a flame to destroy any bacteria.

On collecting a specimen from a female patient a clean bed-pan must be given and she must be asked to avoid having her bowels open at the same time ; should she be menstruating, the vulva is swabbed with a mild cleansing solution, then a small pad of absorbent cotton-wool is placed just inside the vaginal orifice whilst the urine is voided so that no contamination of the specimen from the vagina is possible. When bacteriological examination is required a 'catheter specimen' must be obtained with strict aseptic technique.

Collecting a 24-hour Specimen of Urine.—Whilst the analysis of a single specimen will merely reveal the presence of abnormal constituents, it is only by collecting all the urine that is passed during the 24 hours that a quantitative analysis can be made showing the total amount of each constituent secreted by the kidney throughout the day. Great care must be exercised in the collection in order that all the urine voided in the 24 hours is included and that no extraneous matter is allowed to contaminate it.

In order that the patient may be kept under close supervision it is often more convenient to keep him in bed for the 24 hours. This will reduce the risks of secretive voiding of urine and of specimens being overlooked.

Equipment required, which will be assembled on a tray, will include fluid balance chart, sterile urinal, sterile measure, two Winchester bottles suitably marked with the patient's name, ward, hospital, and date and title of specimen. The bladder should be completely emptied at the time specified for beginning the collection, this urine being discarded. Thereafter, all the urine passed is placed in a dark-glass Winchester bottle which has been specially prepared by the laboratory, the quantity and time of each voiding being noted on the fluid balance chart. At the expiration of the 24 hours the patient is again requested to empty the bladder and this amount is included in the specimen. The whole procedure must be explained to the patient in order that he may co-operate, and every nurse who is likely to have some responsibility in collection should be made familiar with the requirements.

COLLECTION OF BLOOD SPECIMENS

Samples of blood are being investigated on a much larger scale and this tendency is likely to increase as the doctors prescribe more and more drugs and probe still further into the causes of mental subnormality.

A great deal of information concerning the chemical contents of the body becomes available on examination of the blood, as, for example, the isolation of the known ten plasma aminoacidopathies. As the techniques are developed it will be possible to complete most of the known blood investigations using only minute quantities of blood. These possibilities are already being demonstrated successfully.

Requirements.—Although research into this subject is progressing at a rapid pace its effect will only filter through to the majority of hospitals slowly; it will therefore still be necessary for the nurse to continue to carry out the well-established technique of preparing for the collection of a sample of blood.

Disposable sterile syringes (2-, 5-, 10-, or 20-ml.) with a suitable disposable needle will be required, together with the following items : Antiseptic and swabs to cleanse the skin ; tourniquet to compress the vein so that it will stand out prominently and make it easy to insert the needle ; sterile specimen bottles labelled with the patient's name, hospital, and date and time of collection of the specimen.

Some blood specimens are placed in bottles which contain some anticoagulant substance such as citrate, heparin, fluoride, or oxalate, usually for whole-blood or plasma estimations.

The nurse should check with the doctor taking the specimen to find out which type of specimen bottle he requires.

Pathological specimen request forms should be readily available for the doctor to complete and to accompany the specimen.

BONE-MARROW PUNCTURE

Examination of the bone-marrow cells to estimate their chromosome content is a more complicated method and requires a minor surgical procedure.

In adults the sites in which this is usually performed are the iliac crests and the sternum.

A sterile trolley is required containing dressing, towels, skin antiseptic, swabs, 2 per cent procaine hydrochloride with syringe and needles, and a small scalpel. The special narrow-puncture needles together with syringe to fit are usually provided by the laboratory.

Marrow is aspirated from the bone cavity with full aseptic precautions and spread on slides.

BUCCAL SMEARS

The examination of buccal smears is a simple method for collecting material from a patient to study and determine his chromosome constitution.

Requirements.—Adequate lighting in order that the mouth cavity is well illuminated ; spatulæ, usually resembling an ice-cream spoon ; glass slides ; cover slides ; fixative for the buccal smear ; sectionalized container for the slides.

It is the usual procedure for the laboratory technician or doctor to collect their own specimens.

THE ELECTRO-ENCEPHALOGRAM

The electro-encephalogram (E.E.G.) is a record of the electrical activity of the brain, and the machine used to register such activity is the electro-encephalograph. It consists of eight or more identical channels of amplification which are recorded on a continuous paper graph. The cerebral activity is collected by about twenty electrodes, which are small saline pads placed on the head in a symmetrical arrangement according to particular recognized patterns.

For most routine recordings the patient lies quietly on the couch, opening and closing his eyes to command. Other stimuli are usually applied such as overbreathing, which produces slight alkalosis, and intermittent photic stimulation using a very short, high-intensity flash at varying frequencies. These often increase the instability of the E.E.G. and may produce epileptic disturbances that up to this time did not show on records.

One of the main problems of recording the E.E.G. of the mentally subnormal person is the lack of sustained effort in his ability to co-operate.

Greater use is being made of the E.E.G. in an effort to localize causative foci of the brain for behaviour disturbances and epilepsy. In some hospitals this has become a routine investigation following admission, and it is usually necessary to discontinue all drugs for 24 hours preceding the investigation, unless instructions to the contrary have been given. It is often necessary for repeated E.E.G.'s to be taken in order that more and fuller information may be made available to the doctor.

13

CHAPTER XIV

COMMUNITY CARE

COMMUNITY care is a well-used scheme for caring for the mentally subnormal person outside the precincts of the hospital.

The Mental Health Act, 1959, makes fresh provision for the care and treatment of the mentally subnormal, the hope being that more out-patient and community care will be possible for a greater number of patients.

Great efforts are being made to provide a more realistic approach to the problems of community care. Special workshops are being introduced where the patients are employed on a factory basis, ' clocking in ' and ' clocking out ', and are paid on results without the stress of factory competitiveness.

The Ministry of Labour has recognized these workshops as ' sheltered ', thus enabling the patients working in them to be placed on the Disabled Persons' Register with a guarantee of a minimum salary.

Mentally subnormal patients may receive help and training from the government-subsidized Industrial Rehabilitation units. Following satisfactory adjustment to employment, selected patients are then found work in other factories and efforts are made to find suitable lodgings in the community. Already some mental health authorities are preparing plans for the development of small family group hostels where patients who are incapable of adjusting themselves to their home environment or to lodgings, yet do not need the full services of a hospital, can make their home.

Through this enlightened approach and the greater understanding of a sympathetic community which has learnt to accept them, it is hoped that many patients will learn to become self-supporting, independent, and useful members of the community.

With the improved community services and the use of modern drugs it is hoped that many patients will recover from the effects of long institutionalization and, with the exception of the most severe cases, will avoid admission to hospital, which is to be the aim of the future.

Local mental health authorities have a statutory responsibility to provide a mental welfare officer service. In the most recent years a course of training has been made available by most authorities in order that the workers may be trained to do their job successfully and to be able to deal with all the human problems that are likely to come their way.

The responsibilities of the mental welfare officer service will include the care and after-care of the mentally subnormal person in the community, home visiting to offer guidance, advice, and support, and to take an active part in the running of training centres and clubs.

The mental welfare officer works in close co-operation with the general practitioner in the community and the Responsible Medical Officer in the hospital. He is a member of a team which also includes psychiatrists and psychologists, who attend out-patient clinics and hospital case conferences.

Community living for the mentally subnormal person can be a hazardous existence. Because of his low mentality there is a tendency for people to feel that it is not worth helping him.

Four approaches should be thought of when assisting community adjustment.

1. **Morale.**—Being mentally subnormal and not acceptable to the community at large has many problems. Keeping happy in a world of few understandable interests and activities is not easy ; states of depression and conflict must occur.

With the community's increased knowledge of mental subnormality and their growing acceptance of it, it will become a part of our method of living.

A patient who has given up hope, and almost consciously takes on the role of a difficult, unreliable, severely handicapped person, has said goodbye to the development of his potential, to his health, as well as to his happiness and his purpose in life.

2. **Physical Health.**—Hinging on the feeling that no one cares, and hopelessness, is apathy on the patient's part about

safeguarding his health. Four common health hazards facing the patient will concern his hearing, his eyesight, the teeth, and the feet. For remedial treatment to be successful it must be instituted before the state of apathy sets in.

3. **Food.**—Poor feeding will result from ignorance, apathy, and frustration. The main factor in keeping these people well is plenty of good food. For many years now the authorities have seen that young children at school get a good meal and extra milk daily. It is just as essential to see that the mentally subnormal person receives the same amount of nourishment.

4. **Emotional Health.**—There are two important factors which will affect and undermine the emotional stability of a person. These are : (1) Loneliness ; (2) Unemployability.

Life under these conditions becomes a fearful contest between his wilfulness, the community, and his home. The only source from which prevention is available is the local mental health services.

OUT-PATIENT CLINICS

Out-patient clinics are a relatively new development in the care of the mentally subnormal person and are usually held in the out-patient department of a general hospital.

The services they aim to provide include : diagnosis, advice on policies of treatment, the giving of help and advice to harassed anxious parents, counselling, making early admission available for the more urgent cases, and co-ordination of all available services.

One of their primary functions is to support and maintain the patient in his family unit and in the community.

The number of visits and their frequency will depend upon the patient and upon the degree of family adjustment required.

The diagnosis is usually an attempt at going beyond just a clinical level in considering differential diagnosis, aetiological diagnosis, occupational and educational diagnosis of associated medical and emotional findings, and social diagnosis in relation to the family and community. All are equally important and are thoroughly investigated. There is also an attempt to give the family some idea of the child's prognosis.

Parents' counselling is offered to help the parents to understand and to adjust to the problem of having a mentally subnormal child in their family.

Follow-up care is provided in conjunction with the local mental health department. Other facilities available through the clinics are : dental treatment, psychiatric care, speech therapy, physiotherapy, group therapy, play therapy, and occupational and recreational therapy.

The values of out-patient clinics are :—

1. They offer a team approach in the evaluation of a full diagnostic approach to the patient, which is essential for planning the kind of care, training, and services required by the patient and his family. The facilities offer adequate time for parent counselling at the same time as dealing with the child.

2. They are places where the parents can gain sorely needed help and advice without having to pass from one source of disappointment and disillusion to another.

3. They permit easier access to the hospital service if this is found to be urgent.

TRAINING CENTRES FOR CHILDREN AND HOME TEACHING

The provision of some form of alternative training for mentally subnormal children and adults who are unable to benefit from the normal education system is regarded as an essential feature of a modern mental health service.

The mentally subnormal require training and occupation to replace the normal activities of school and employment from which they are generally barred, and to ' educate ' them in the widest sense to live as social beings within the small circle of their immediate family and the wider group of the whole community.

Home visits and other assistance provided by the mental health social worker are not sufficient on their own to meet fully the social needs of the mentally handicapped person who lives at home with his family.

The training centre provides a service in the community which meets this dual need of the family and the subnormal person simultaneously. It provides training and occupation, to keep him alert and happy and to develop his latent faculties, and it offers the family some welcome relief from the strain involved in his day-to-day care and management at home. Looking after a severely mentally subnormal person continuously is demanding in responsibility, emotionally and physically; without some relief it can produce nervous strain and domestic and family friction.

Having her child accepted by the training centre and knowing that other people are prepared to look after him for some hours has the effect of making the mother more relaxed, and it helps her to build up her self-respect. The experience of meeting other parents with children attending the centre is valuable, as she may discover that her own problems, which may seem insurmountable, are shared by others and are being conquered.

The advantages that the child derives from attending a training centre are numerous. First of all he has the prestige of attending school and travelling by coach. Instead of being left at home all day, feeling lonely, different, frustrated, and unable to join in play-groups with other children, he has a special place of his own to go to with children who have the same limitations as his own. He is able to join in their activities and he may possibly excel as a leader. At the centre he can produce things to show off at home, which are as much to be prized by his family as the awards that the normal members may bring home. The key work of the centre is to help the mentally subnormal to become socially acceptable despite his disabilities, his unusual appearance, his lack of speed and physical awkwardness. Through careful training matched by his needs and by the stimulus derived from competing within a group which has his handicap too, much of his social skill is achieved.

Remedial exercises, speech therapy, handicrafts, music and singing, free play, and the sharing of small responsibilities and duties, all play their part in the training scheme, reinforced implicitly by the example of tolerance and patience shown by the teachers and nurses.

A teacher can often achieve more obvious results than the parents because she will have him for a limited time only and her entire store of energy is available to meet his needs.

Home Teaching.—In some rural districts, where there are mentally handicapped people scattered over large areas, and where transport difficulties make it impossible for them to be collected and taken to a centre, home teaching is provided in lieu of a centre. It is, however, a poor substitute. Parents are given the feeling that the child is getting some help. The visits of the teacher afford the mother the opportunity of talking over the child's problems with someone who understands some of the difficulties.

CLUBS

Some voluntary bodies, with the financial assistance and moral support of their local health, education, and youth departments provide club facilities for all mentally subnormal patients living in the community.

It is usually necessary for the club to be sited in a central area so that patients from all corners of the district can reach it with reasonable comfort, using the public transport. It may be necessary for club transport and transport hostesses to be made available for taking any physically handicapped members to and from the club.

The club building must be capable of being functional for all the variety of needs of the members. It must be accessible from the main road and the entrance must be free from steps or severe slopes. Doorways should be wide enough to allow wheel chairs to pass through. Toilets and wash-hand basins should be adequate and on ground level; all the main rooms and kitchen should also be on ground level in order to avoid the necessity of physical transportation of patients up and down flights of stairs.

The club should be run as far as possible on normal lines, so that the patients are treated as though they were normal.

The role of the social worker in such a setting can be a vital one, particularly with ex-hospital patients who are gaining new social experiences and self-confidence, and who are in need of help to form new relationships with new groups, and introductions to the church and other community groups which may be helpful to them. These continuing programmes are even more important when the patient lacks supporting relatives or helpful friends. For the recently discharged hospital patient, clubs can help to bridge the gap between hospital and the outside world.

MENTAL HEALTH SOCIAL WORKERS

This is a service provided by the hospital management committees, and the mental health social worker is becoming more and more an important member of the hospital team whose primary function is social case work in the hospital and community. She is trained to understand and handle personal and social problems related to the mentally subnormal person, his parents, and the community. The social worker's contribution as a member of the team is primarily directed towards the rehabilitation and after-care of the patient. She helps the patient to face and overcome the problems which arise from having been isolated in hospital for long periods. She helps the patient to help himself and endeavours to consolidate the training given in the hospital.

In her work the social worker is looked upon as a friend and adviser of the patient, his relatives, and, in some cases, his employer.

To be successful she must have a wide knowledge of all the available social services and how to obtain help from them.

The social worker is the person who presents the doctor with a social history and family background of the patient. She is the liaison officer between the hospital and the community, the family doctor and the local mental health authority.

Arranging after-care, rehabilitation, suitable employment, or special training takes up much of the social worker's time.

She needs to have a desire to help humanity, to have a sincere sensitive understanding of people, and to be an expert in interpersonal relationships.

DAY WORK

Day work is the terminal phase in the rehabilitation programme, when a patient is employed in the community but continues to be resident in the hospital.

A hospital 'community rehabilitation' programme, even the best conceived and most expertly implemented, cannot fully meet the requirements of those patients whose prognosis indicates the probable return to community living. Although the hospital work may in every respect try to replicate similar work situations in the community, there are certain essential ingredients which are not present in the hospital setting. All workshop supervisors in a hospital are aware of and usually considerate of the patient's handicap; although the staff may be concerned with production and with fulfilling their contracts they have some understanding of the patient's limitations and take these into account in their interpersonal relationships. On this kind of programme there is no possibility for him to experience being sacked. If his adjustment is not satisfactory or if he is unable to perform his work adequately he is transferred to another type of work. Unlike people in the community he does not have the opportunity to earn to the extent of being self-supporting. Though he does earn it is usually only a token amount and will provide only for weekly pocket-money requirements.

Experiences such as using public transport, public recreational facilities, and the experience of purchasing personal requirements in the local stores are absent.

Group activities which have been planned for the hospital patients do not provide opportunities for individual choice in the way that industrial recreation clubs do.

Day work can be utilized to evaluate the patient's skills in a real job situation and can provide experiences in different kinds of occupations. Its most important value lies in its potential to shorten the overall hospital experience of the patient, providing him with an opportunity to develop confidence in his own abilities and the positive sense of achievement and satisfaction when receiving his weekly pay-packet.

The patient will need considerable support, guidance, and encouragement in the early days in order to overcome the many problems and difficulties which he is certain to meet. These will include a discipline prepared for normal people, interpersonal relationships with his foreman and work colleagues, the impersonal factory environment, lack of experience in the use of the community's services, handling relatively large amounts of money, and budgeting for a week at a time.

DANGERS OF COMMUNITY CARE

On his return to community life the patient may have a feeling of anxiety, because he is in a strange environment, living with people who have a better living skill than he has, and his inferiority is impressed upon him by his inability to keep up to the standards of those in his immediate surroundings. Unless he is given a true feeling of security he will fail to adjust himself to communal living.

The parents' attitude towards the patient can be one of over-indulgence, rejection, or acceptance with understanding.

In the first case, the parents feel they must do everything for their child, take every precaution against frustrations, and meet every need without delay. If the patient has been discharged from hospital he has some power of self-care which will continue, providing the necessary stimulus and training continue, but he will be only too pleased to relinquish his independence if people are prepared to save him the trouble of personal effort. Mentally subnormal patients, like children, quickly recognize a slackening of authority and as quickly take their opportunity of gaining control of those caring for them. The over-indulgent parent will make the patient a helpless, dependent, and difficult person. Constancy in attitude and management is an important factor not to be overlooked by parent, guardian, or nurse. Over-anxiety or over-ambition will produce emotional difficulties equal to those produced by uninterested neglect.

In the second case, that of rejection, patients quickly sense their unwantedness and the opposition of society and as a result their protective mechanism comes into play. They build around themselves a grandiose personality and develop antisocial behaviour which will quickly lead them into trouble. In the home the parents must accept the patient as one of the family.

The most satisfactory parents are those who understand the patient, are prepared to accept him and make him welcome, but are not prepared to allow him to gain control over them. A community educated to the understanding of the mentally subnormal will in most cases accept him as one of themselves and will not expect too much from him.

The risks involved in discharging a mentally subnormal person to community care may arise from a period of enforced idleness owing to his lack of adaptability. He must be kept fully occupied for the entire day.

Also in his daily work it is more than likely that the patient will have to work beside a person of average intelligence, whose working capacity will far exceed that of the mentally subnormal. Allowance must be made for this. Criticism must be cut to the minimum, and then it should only be constructive and made in such a manner as not to discourage the patient.

Lack of control over mentally subnormal persons may encourage insolent and unruly behaviour. The cause of the behaviour must first be isolated and where possible remedied. In cases where the cause is obscure and the patient refuses to co-operate hospitalization becomes necessary.

Marriage and the Procreation of Children.—Marriage between mentally subnormal patients is not illegal, but it is not desirable. Marriages do occur and not all of them are unsuccessful, though usually the couple require a great deal of guidance and supervision in managing their lives. The great disadvantage is the risk that any off-spring of the union may be mentally subnormal, but it may, of course, produce normal children. Frequent talks, simply given, will be necessary before it can be felt that the patient has at least some understanding of the responsibilities of marriage.

Social Misbehaviour.—Mentally subnormal patients are not more highly sexed than the normal person ; indeed, they may possess less sex energy, but owing to lack of will-power and control they demonstrate the channels along which their minds are running. Indecent exposure and interference with young children are the most serious offences. This would rarely happen if the mentally subnormal person were kept occupied and correctly supervised by the parent and social worker. Vetting of literature and films is valuable in order that erotic stimuli may be avoided.

Unscrupulous Exploitation.—The unsupervised, disheartened, and disinterested patient is an easy tool in the hands of people wanting to make use of the weak-minded person.

There are still employers who will not recognize that mentally subnormal persons must have time off from work for relaxation. They tend to overwork patients, who, because they have not the ability to protest through the normal channels, may take the law into their own hands and either run away or steal or become aggressive.

Education of the Parent or Guardian of a Discharged Patient.—One of the best ways of overcoming a difficult problem is by a parents' association through which parents can discuss their problems with each other. There will be a great need for advice and encouragement which no one else but the doctor, nurse, and social worker will be in a position to give. It must be impressed upon parents or guardians that in order to keep a patient happy he must be in full occupation with a varied curriculum, and encouraged to be independent of others. The dangers of monotony, boredom, and frustration must be guarded against. Whilst the mentally subnormal person is in hospital he is one among many people in a similar condition. His contacts are with those having the same restrictions and his own shortcomings are therefore not conspicuous. In the community, however, he is the odd man out, and his restricted capacities are easily noticeable.

CHAPTER XV

DRUGS AND THEIR INDICATIONS

It is useful for nurses to have an elementary knowledge of the commoner drugs in use, both as regards their indications, dosage and possible side-reactions. The drugs in common use are conveniently divided into certain classes, according to the prominent action produced by them. The list included here is by no means complete as the science of pharmacology is constantly producing new drugs of every kind.

In the light of experience drugs once thought to be free from any serious side reactions are now found to be serious in their effect on the human body when taken in continuous treatment. The classes of drugs included here and considered to be part of the essential knowledge of the nurse are :—

1. Sedatives (*Table I*).
2. Anticonvulsants (*Table II*).
3. Antispasmodics (*Table III*).
4. Stimulants (*Table IV*).
5. Tranquillizers (*Table V*).
6. Antidepressants (*Table VI*).
7. Miscellaneous (*Table VII*).

More Recent Drugs in Use for Mental Illness.— During the last 15 years there has been a rapid growth in the number and types of drugs made available for the treatment of all forms of mental illness. They have brought about a great breakthrough of the barrier of psychiatric disorders.

For clinical practice these drugs have been classified into groups. The three main groups are :—

1. Tranquillizers or neuroleptics.
2. Antidepressants or thymoleptics.
3. Miscellaneous group.

Table I.—SEDATIVES

DRUG (*Barbiturates*)	TRADE NAME	AVERAGE DAILY DOSE	INDICATIONS	SIDE REACTIONS	NURSING CARE
Long Action Barbitone sodium	Medinal Veronal sodium	300–600 mg.	Sleeplessness (with analgesics for relief of pain)	Cumulative action (use over long period may produce mental and moral changes with depressive tendencies, pathological changes in the central nervous system)	Antidote—picrotoxin. Artificial respiration + oxygen Aim to maintain respiration and eliminate the drug Treatment for over-dosage: stomach lavage leaving amphetamine sulphate in stomach if patient is comatosed
Phenobarbitone	Gardenal Luminal	30–120 mg.	Epilepsy, sleeplessness	As for barbitone sodium	As for barbitone sodium. Sudden withdrawal from epileptic patient may lead to relapse
Methylphenobarbitone	Prominal	60–200 mg.	Epilepsy	As for barbitone sodium	As for barbitone sodium
Intermediate Action Amylobarbitone	Amytal	100–200 mg.	Sleeplessness, epilepsy, and anxiety states	As for barbitone sodium	As for barbitone sodium
Butobarbitone	Soneryl	100–200 mg. Maximum dose in 24 hr. 360 mg.	Insomnia and nervous conditions	As for barbitone sodium	As for barbitone sodium

DRUG (Barbiturates)	TRADE NAME	AVERAGE DAILY DOSE	INDICATIONS	SIDE REACTIONS	NURSING CARE
Short Action					
Cyclobarbitone	Phanodorm	200–400 mg.	Insomnia and anxiety states	As for barbitone sodium	As for barbitone sodium
Pentobarbitone sodium	Nembutal	100–200 mg.	Acute anxiety states prior to inhalation anaesthesia	As for barbitone sodium	As for barbitone sodium
Quinalbarbitone sodium	Seconal	150–200 mg.	Insomnia and anxiety states	As for barbitone sodium	As for barbitone sodium
Chloral hydrate		0·3–2 g.	Nervous insomnia, mania		Must be given as a mixture well diluted; withdraw from patient gradually. For over-dosage: gastric lavage using 2 gallons of water; keep patient roused but at rest and warm. Nikethamide and stimulants
Paraldehyde		2–7 ml.	To quieten and induce sleep in the mentally disordered	Erythematous rash, gastric irritation. May cause toxic hepatitis	Avoid administration over long periods because of addiction. For over-dosage: gastric lavage or emetic strychnine 8 mg. hypodermically. Nikethamide; methylamphetamine. Artificial respiration
Mephenesin sedative	Myanesin	0·5–1·0 g. one to six times daily by mouth	Spastic hypertonic, hyperkinetic conditions	Slight nausea and drowsiness	Antidote—intubate patient and institute controlled respiration. Treat severe fall in blood-pressure with methylamphetamine hydrochloride

Table II.—Anticonvulsants

Drug	Trade Name	Average Daily Dose	Indications	Side Reactions	Nursing Care
Acetazolamide	Diamox	375–1000 mg. daily in divided doses	Epilepsy	Drowsiness, paresthesia, fatigue, excitement, gastro-intestinal upsets, disorientation, agranulocytosis	Frequent blood count
Methoin	Mesontoin	100–600 mg.	Epilepsy—grand mal	Dermatitis, agranulocytosis, aplastic anaemia	Frequent blood count
Paramethadione	Paradione	Adults and older children 600–900 mg.	Epilepsy—petit mal	General rashes, depression of bone-marrow	Weekly blood count
Phenytoin sodium	Epanutin Eptoin	50–200 mg.	Epilepsy—grand mal	Sickness, nausea, dizziness, skin rashes, tremors, fevers, mental confusion, hallucinations, dermatitis, gastric irritation	If a patient is taking barbiturates or bromides, transfer to this drug should be made gradually
Primidone	Mysoline	Adults: 0·5–2 g. Children: 0·25–1·0 g. in divided doses	Epilepsy	Mild and transitory giddiness, nausea, and vomiting. Occasionally megaloblastic anaemia	15 mg. folic acid daily for megaloblastic anaemia
Sulthiame	Ospolot	50–200 mg.	Epilepsy — grand mal, with behaviour disorders, temporal lobe epilepsy, Jacksonian seizures, myoclonic seizures, hyperkinetic behaviour	Parasthesia of the face and extremities, tachypnoea, dyspnoea, headache, giddiness, ataxia, anorexia, nausea, loss of weight	
Troxidonum	Tridione	Adults: 900 mg.–1·8 g. Children: 2–5 yr., 300–900 mg. daily; 6–12 yr. 600–	Epilepsy—petit mal	Hepatitis, visual disturbance, rashes, anaemia, agranulocytosis	Weekly blood counts; as treatment progresses, monthly

Table III.—ANTISPASMODICS

DRUG	TRADE NAME	AVERAGE DAILY DOSE	INDICATIONS	SIDE REACTIONS	NURSING CARE
Atropine sulphate		0·25–2 mg. maximum dose in 24 hrs. by mouth	Post-encephalitic Parkinsonism, poisoning by morphine	Dryness of mouth, burning sensation in throat	The antidote is 1·3 g. of ac. tannic in 118 ml. of water followed by an emetic. Short-acting barbiturates given intravenously. General symptoms are relieved by pilocarpine 5 mg. at repeated intervals. Give plenty of fluid
Belladonna (tincture)		0·5–2 ml.	Post-encephalitic Parkinsonism	As for atropine	Antidote as for atropine
Benzhexol hydrochloride (synthetic drug)	Artane	2–20 mg. in divided doses	Post-encephalitic or arteriosclerotic Parkinsonism	Dryness of mouth, nausea, and vomiting	Treatment should never be terminated suddenly
Stramonium (tincture)		0·5–2 ml. in Parkinsonism	Post-encephalitic Parkinsonism	As for atropine	Antidote as for atropine

Table IV.—STIMULANTS

Drug	Trade Name	Average Daily Dose	Indications	Side Reactions	Nursing Care
Amphetamine sulphate	Benzedrine	2·5–10 mg.	Narcolepsy, post-encephalitic Parkinsonism, mild depressive neuroses, barbiturate poisoning	Mouth dryness, restlessness, insomnia, anorexia. *Large doses*: cardiovascular reactions, convulsions, coma. Do not give at same time as, or within 21 days of ceasing, monoamine oxidase inhibitors	Addiction frequent. Antidote—a rapidly acting barbiturate by injection, or cyclobarbitone, quinalbarbitone, orally
Dexamphetamine sulphate	Dexedrine	5–10 mg.	As for amphetamine sulphate, effective in smaller doses		
Methylamphetamine hydrochloride	Methedrine	2·5–10 mg. orally. 10–30 mg. by injection	As for amphetamine sulphate, more rapid in effect, lasts for longer period, but is more toxic		

Drug	Trade Name	Average Daily Dose	Indications	Side Reactions	Nursing Care	Remarks
Chlorpromazine	Largactil	75–500 mg. orally daily. 25–50 mg. by injection, repeated as required three or four times in 24 hours	Excitement or extreme agitation in organic psychosis, mental tension, excitable states in the mentally subnormal person	Drowsiness, hypotension, Parkinsonism, dry mouth, jaundice	Observe for the appearance of any side reactions and for the appearance of skin disorders. The nurse must take precautions and not handle the drug unless she is wearing rubber gloves. Regular blood count	Patients must be kept in supine position for at least 1 hr. after injection
Thioridazine	Melleril	30–600 mg. daily	Neurosis and psychosis	Drowsiness, dizziness, faintness, dryness of mouth, transient œdema		
Promazine hydrochloride	Sparine	800 mg. 25–200 mg. one to four times daily	Useful in alcoholism due to the absence of toxic effects on the liver. Excitable states and agitation	Blood dycrasias, hypotension, tremors		
Acepromazine	Notensil	75 mg. in three divided doses	Excitable states and agitation			
Prochlorperazine	Stemetil Compozine	15–30 mg.	Dizziness and vertigo sickness	Parkinsonism, restlessness		
Haloperidol	Serenace	1·5–10 mg. daily	Psychotic disorders	Parkinsonism		Caution if giving to hysterical patients

*Table V.—*TRANQUILLIZERS *(Contd.)*

DRUG	TRADE NAME	AVERAGE DAILY DOSE	INDICATIONS	SIDE REACTIONS	NURSING CARE	REMARKS
Fluphenazine	Moditen	1–5 mg. daily	As for chlorpromazine	As for chlorpromazine	Watch for extra-pyramidal symptoms	
Fluphenazine cenenthane injection	Moditen	25 mg. every 2 or 3 weeks intramuscular	As for chlorpromazine	As for chlorpromazine	Watch for extra-pyramidal symptoms	
Perphenazine	Fentazin Trilofon	8–24 mg.	Anxiety and agitated and excited patients	Tonic neck contractions, trismus		More potent and less toxic than Largactil. Patients suffering from leucopenia should not be given this drug
Trifluoperazine	Stelazine	Mild cases 2–4 mg. daily. Chronic or acute cases 15–30 mg. daily	Aggression and excitability	Agranulocytosis	Regular blood count	Ten times more potent than Largactil. A popular drug for the treatment of aggression
Reserpine	Serpasil	1–5 mg. daily in divided doses	Useful in the treatment of the psychotic	Severe depression, fall in body temperature, low blood-pressure, salivation, Parkinsonism	Discontinue reserpine for at least 7 days before E.C.T.	

Table VI.—ANTIDEPRESSANTS

DRUG	TRADE NAME	AVERAGE DAILY DOSE	INDICATIONS	SIDE REACTIONS	NURSING CARE	REMARKS
Phenelzine di-hydrogen sulphate	Nardil	45 mg.	Mild depression	Œdema, hypotension, nausea		A monoamine oxidase inhibitor
Nialamide	Niamid	25–150 mg.	Mild depression	Dry mouth, sweating, dizziness, blurred vision		A monoamine oxidase inhibitor
Isocarboxazid	Marplan	40 mg.	Mild depression, angina pectoris, agitation	Coryza-like symptoms, œdema, hypotension, vertigo		A monoamine oxidase inhibitor
Imipramine	Tofranil	Up to 150 mg.	Severe depression, sleeplessness associated with manic-depressive states	Dry mouth, œdema, pruritus, hypotension		This is not a monoamine oxidase inhibitor
Tranylcypromine	Parnate	20 mg.	Severe depression	Restlessness, dizziness, dry mouth, headache, agitation	Signs of overdosage are excitability, hyperpyrexia, collapse. Treat the condition by administering a gastric lavage. Promazine is the antidote	A monoamine oxidase inhibitor

Table VII.—Miscellaneous Group

Drug	Trade Name	Average Daily Dose	Indications	Side Reactions	Nursing Care
Chlordiazepoxide	Librium	30–100 mg.	Tension, anxiety, functional disorders, agitation, phobias, obsessions	Ataxia, drowsiness, nausea, constipation	Regular attention to the bowels in order to avoid severe constipation
Chlorprothixene	Taractan	30–600 mg.	Behaviour disorders, agitated depression, manic depressive psychoses	Orthostatic hypotension, tachycardia, Parkinsonism	
Diazepam	Valium	4–40 mg. daily in divided doses	Tension, anxiety, epilepsy, neuroses, psychoses		

Tranquillizers.—These drugs are used on the disturbed patient and produce calmness without affecting clearness of consciousness.

It is important that the nurses who are responsible for the administration of this group of drugs should be familiar with the side reactions and toxic effects so that they may recognize their onset and take immediate action to counteract them.

Antidepressants.—These drugs primarily affect the patient's mood. The monoamine oxidase inhibitors inhibit or suppress enzymes in the brain which normally destroy the amines. The use of these drugs leads to biochemical changes in the central nervous system. There is usually a period of 7–21 days following the first administration of the drug before any clinical effect can be expected and it may be that during this period there will be serious deterioration of the patient's mental condition.

Again, it is important for the nurse to be aware of the possible side reactions, such as hypotension and severe mood swings.

The antidepressant drugs are used in the treatment of depression, but electroconvulsive therapy still remains the treatment of choice in severe depression.

Miscellaneous.—These drugs are used for the sympathetic relief of anxiety and tension. They are relatively new drugs and not a lot is known of their true clinical value or of their side reactions, and it is therefore important that the nurse observes her patients very carefully and makes careful notes on her observations.

New drugs of these types are introduced from time to time.

CHAPTER XVI

MENTAL ILLNESS
IN RELATION TO MENTAL SUBNORMALITY

MOST mental illnesses do not show themselves until after the adolescent stage has been reached, compared with mental subnormality, which occurs with the beginning of life or soon after. In mental illness there has been a fully developed mind which has become feeble, whereas in mental subnormality it has never been fully developed.

Though the sufferers from some mental illnesses may appear mentally subnormal, they may be distinguished by the presence of delusions, hallucinations, and impulsive conduct. These patients tend to get worse, but may have periods when they appear to have slightly improved. Many have specific treatments.

Mental illness can be discussed under two headings :—
Mental illness associated with mental subnormality.
Mental illness superimposed on mental subnormality.

MENTAL ILLNESS ASSOCIATED WITH
MENTAL SUBNORMALITY

There are two different types of mental illness which must be considered : those which create a picture similar to mental subnormality ; and those which may make a subnormal more subnormal.

The mental illnesses which are akin to mental subnormality are :—

1. Schizophrenia.
2. Toxic psychoses.
3. Dementia.

1. **Schizophrenia.**—This is a condition in which there is a gradual disintegration of the personality. There is often a

hereditary tendency, the patient coming from neurotic stock, but environmental factors have a bearing on the incidence and there is some evidence to suggest that the condition may be due to biochemical abnormality.

It has been described as an attempt by the individual to 'make the unlivable livable'.

It was once regarded as hopelessly incurable but now there is cause for greater optimism in many cases, though some still make a rapid progress towards a chronic weak-mindedness.

Schizophrenia requires a schizoid type of temperament in which to develop, this being characterized by reticence, aloof-ness, partial divorcement from reality, and an inability to adapt to changing circumstances and to make personal contact.

Schizophrenic illnesses are frequently classified into four types, and all four may show the characteristics of each other. The major features of the illness are : severe thought disorder, fantastic and grotesque delusions, vivid hallucinations, tenden-cies to stereotyped movements, stupor alternating with frenzy, impulsive violence and suicide, and a disharmony between mood and thought.

The four schizophrenic illnesses are :—

a. Simple Schizophrenia.—This disorder usually develops during adolescence or early adulthood. It has an insidious onset, its only manifestation being a lack of drive, an odd manner, and a lack of emotional tone. There is a gradual personality change towards a disharmony between mood and thought and towards eccentricity. Later in the course of the disease various delusions may occur. Hallucinations may be present and some patients exhibit antisocial tendencies such as stealing and indecent exposure.

b. Hebephrenic Schizophrenia.—This is a disorder which affects young people ; the onset is acute. Hallucinations are very common, the patient being preoccupied with his voices, often smiling or giggling to himself. Delusions occur which produce foolish erratic behaviour accompanied by mannerisms and strange antics. The illness tends to be progressive and even temporary recovery is unusual.

c. Paranoid Schizophrenia.—This disorder begins later in life, usually between 30 and 40 years of age. It is characterized by paranoid type delusions; hallucinations and thought disturbance may be present also. The delusions are of a persecutory and grandiose nature. The patient very often claims that he is being influenced by hypnotism and that his mind and body are being controlled by various forces such as machinery and electricity. He may complain that his mind is being read or that he has been sexually assaulted.

With the use of tranquillizing drugs the prognosis is more hopeful.

d. Catatonic Schizophrenia.—This disorder has a more abrupt onset than the other three states and recovery is more likely to occur. The onset is acute and almost without warning, and there are two distinct phases :—

i. *Stupor* : This is a state of rigid immobility. The patient sits or stands in various attitudes. He may be mute or repeat what is said to him ; mannerisms are common. Consciousness is not lost and memory is preserved.

ii. *Excitement* : The patient displays absurd behaviour which is stereotyped, purposeless, and often violent and impulsive. Speech is confused and incoherent, and there is a lack of emotional tone. The habits may be filthy and degraded. Hallucinations may be present.

2. Toxic Psychoses.—Mental disturbances appear as a result of the presence of toxic bodies, drugs, chemicals, fatigue, or illness. In this book our concern lies with the mental disturbances caused by the barbiturate drugs. When taken in excess they give rise to delirium, confusion, ataxy of speech and gait, constipation, foul breath, and acneiform skin eruptions. Coma may supervene with dilated inactive pupils.

The treatment should consist of : Discontinuation of the drug ; washing out the stomach ; introduction of strong black coffee by a tube ; subcutaneous injection of caffeine and strychnine ; lumbar puncture.

3. Dementia.—The two dementias not already described are :—

a. Pre-senile dementia.

b. Senile dementia.

a. Pre-senile Dementia.—This condition does not normally arise before the age of 18 years, though a man of 30 may be afflicted and may appear to be mentally subnormal.

It occurs as a specific disease which causes deterioration of the brain. There are three main types :—

  i. Pick's disease.
  ii. Alzheimer's disease.
  iii. Huntington's chorea.

  i. *Pick's disease* (circumscribed cortical atrophy) : Atrophic areas develop symmetrically situated in both cortical hemispheres of the frontal and temporal lobes. Mental deterioration is progressive with speech disorder being a striking feature.

  ii. *Alzheimer's disease* : A rare form of cerebral degeneration, the cause of which is unknown.

Physical signs are twitchings and tremors, and convulsions sometimes occur. The limbs are spastic and the patient becomes wasted and bedridden.

Mental symptoms are well marked and progress rapidly. Speech becomes incoherent ; there is loss of memory ; deterioration of habits ; severe disorientation.

  iii. *Huntington's chorea* : This condition is a directly transmitted hereditary condition in which there are degenerative changes in the frontal areas and in the basal ganglia of the cerebrum. Fifty per cent of the children of an affected parent are likely to inherit the condition. Jerky choreiform movements of the face and upper limbs appear early in the disease and are followed by involvement of speech and gait which is ataxic. There is an emotional instability with outbursts of irritability and progressive intellectual deterioration.

The condition progresses for from 10 to 20 years.

b. Senile Dementia.—This is a gradual decay of the bodily and mental functions of a person and is a natural stage of development towards death.

The age at which the bodily and mental powers deteriorate varies greatly with different individuals. One man may be unimpaired at 80, where another is old at 60.

Physical signs : There is usually impairment of health and atrophic wrinkled inelastic skin which often becomes pigmented. The bearing becomes bent and the gait slug-gish. The sensations of hearing and seeing deteriorate.

Mental symptoms : The patient is unable to adapt himself to changes. There is loss of memory for recent happenings, but an easy recall of happenings when young. Delusions and hallucinations may occur. Confusion and disorientation are often present. Deterioration in the patient's mental condition may lead to unclean and degraded habits and he may even be unable to feed himself. Poverty of movement in these patients often leads to chest complications. The prognosis for these patients is one of progressive dementia.

MENTAL ILLNESS SUPERIMPOSED ON MENTAL SUBNORMALITY

The commonest of these mental illnesses are :—

1. Psychotic.
   a. Manic depressive psychosis.
   b. Schizophrenia.
2. Psychoneurotic.
   a. Hysteria.
   b. Anxiety neurosis.
   c. Depression.
3. Psychopathic disorders.
   a. Aggressive.
   b. Inadequate.
   c. Creative.

1. Superimposed Psychosis.—

a. Manic Depressive Psychosis.—The signs and symptoms of this illness are the same in the mentally subnormal as in the normal person, though because of the subnormality some of the symptoms may be less obvious.

Manic depressive psychosis is characterized by sustained swings of mood from elation to depression ; it is in fact an exaggerated version of cyclothymia, a condition found in many normal people.

It is a constitutional illness associated with the pyknic build and may be found to affect other members of the family in varying degrees.

b. Schizophrenia.—

Simple schizophrenia : This disease can masquerade as mental subnormality, but it can usually be isolated because of the delusions which accompany it.

Paranoid schizophrenia : When a normal person becomes afflicted with this condition the disease shows itself as a well-planned and complicated delusion, resembling a complicated murder story where the murderer is trying to cover up his escape.

CYCLOTHYMIA

Mania	*Depression*
Over-active and elated	Slowed up. Apathetic
Over-talkative (garrulous)	Complains of sadness and low spirits
Flight of ideas	Poverty of ideas
Distractability	Apathy
Loss of appetite	Loss of appetite
Too excited to eat	Does not want to eat
Agitation	Agitation in some cases
Loss of weight	Loss of weight
Bizarre, grandiose ideas	Morbid hypochondriacal, suicidal attempts, and self-reproach

Paranoid schizophrenia does occur in mentally subnormal persons, but because of their childish mentality the delusions are less complicated, the scheme of them being more like a child's game.

2. Superimposed Psychoneurosis.—

a. Hysteria.—Hysterical behaviour is a reaction to some difficulty by which the patient is confronted and which he finds hard to overcome. His reaction or motive is resultant upon a cause which is stimulated at the level of the unconscious mind.

Most people are liable to show some sort of hysterical reaction at some period of their lives, but in some these reactions are more severe and persistent ; indeed, they may recur so frequently as to be characteristic of their behaviour.

It is suggested that the hysterical personality is produced by the psychopathology of the childhood background, such as upbringing and environment.

The *symptoms* are egocentric. The person thinks that the world revolves around him. He has shallow feelings for other people though his feelings for himself are deep. Regression to a much earlier age-group is common, e.g., when he refuses to eat and has temper tantrums. If he works he has difficulty in holding down jobs. He prefers immediate gratification of his wishes to distant planning. For example, he would prefer to take a post as ward orderly because of its immediate monetary rewards than pass through the stages of studentship with its prospect of greater rewards in the future.

Two main types of reaction may occur in hysteria :—
  i. Conversion reactions.
  ii. Dissociative reactions.

  i. *Conversion reactions* : This person, after a period of stress and uncertainty, may suddenly develop a paralysis of a limb or any other part of the body which does not correspond with the distribution of the nerves. On examination no abnormality can be found to account for the paralysis.

The symptoms serve a valuable purpose in making a decision over an important problem unnecessary for the patient.

Hysterical prolongation of physical illness is a common malady amongst the mentally subnormal who are given work to do which is too demanding and at the same time makes them feel incompetent and inferior ; because they themselves are conscientious they will become accident prone, and after an accident the injury, in spite of all the treatment and rest, does not improve until the cause of the prolongation of it is removed.

  ii. *Dissociative reactions* : There is a disturbance of consciousness, such as amnesia, fugues, multiple personality, etc.

  b. Anxiety Neurosis.—Anxiety is usually aroused by some threat to the well-being of the individual or by something that threatens to prevent him accomplishing what he wants. It may vary in degree from a mild uneasiness to a terrifying fear.

Only rarely is anxiety neurosis found amongst the mentally subnormal. When it is found it is because that particular patient has a reasonably good personality and a degree of insight. If this patient is given work to do which is too demanding, he will get into a state of anxiety which is a symptom of fear.

The bodily *symptoms* may affect all the systems in the same way that the sympathetic nervous system does during times of stress. These are :—

    i. Rapid pulse (tachycardia).
   ii. Palpitation.
  iii. Irregular breathing.
   iv. Nausea and vomiting.
    v. Griping colicky pains of the bowel.
   vi. Loose stools.
  vii. Tremors of the tongue and hands.
 viii. Feeling of weakness.
   ix. Frequency of micturition.
    x. Sweating.
   xi. Enlargement of the thyroid gland with resulting hyperthyroidism.

The symptoms tend to attract the patient's thoughts to his own bodily functions, and because of this he is liable to develop fears that such a condition as a mild gastric disturbance is an indication of malignancy.

c. Depression.—Reactive exogenous or psychoneurotic depression is a reaction to some external cause, e.g., death of a near relative or the receipt of bad news, but it is more intense or prolonged than one would normally expect.

3. Psychopathic Disorders.—There are three types :—

a. Aggressive.
b. Inadequate.
c. Creative.

a. Aggressive Psychopathic Disorder.—This classification covers the popular conception of the ' cosh boy '. Some of these patients develop this condition as a result of unstable heredity ; unstable environment ; abnormal function of the nervous system.

Signs and *symptoms* are as follows. This patient has no feelings for other people, he is self-centred, and raises no barrier to satisfying his own basic instinctive needs. He has little capacity for forethought and prefers to have immediate fulfilment of his wishes, regardless of the consequences either to himself or anyone else. He has episodic attacks of violence towards other people, the act of violence being much greater than the causative stimulus; for example, rendering an aged person unconscious because he accidentally obstructs his path.

b. *Inadequate Psychopathic Disorder.*—This person is a drifter, moving from place to place and frequently changing his job. This condition is common amongst the subnormals.

Signs and *symptoms* are: No feeling for other people; no interests; the patient is quarrelsome and difficult to manage; very demanding; and very pretentious, claiming that he is more important than he actually is.

c. *Creative Psychopathic Disorder.*—Though this person is unstable he has an artistic temperament displayed either in art or music. He has no feeling for other people.

CHAPTER XVII

METHODS OF TREATMENT

MODIFIED INSULIN THERAPY

This form of treatment is used with great success in patients suffering from neuroses who show symptoms of anxiety and depression, and feelings of tension associated with loss of weight.

The dosage of insulin starts at 10 units and is gradually increased daily to between 60 and 100 units so that the stages of excitement, hypoglycæmia, and coma are avoided. This treatment commences with an intramuscular injection of insulin at 7.30 a.m. and is interrupted at 10 a.m., for 6 days a week, Sunday being a rest day.

Up to 30 treatments are usually given ; this number does vary according to the type of patient being treated and the doctor's assessment of the patient's requirements.

Interruption is effected by giving tea with 20 g. of glucose, immediately followed by a high carbohydrate diet.

The weight usually increases along with the appetite, which may have a psychological beneficial effect on the patient. The insulin also has a mild sedative effect.

ELECTROCONVULSIVE THERAPY (E.C.T.)

This is a form of convulsive therapy which is produced by passing an electrical current through two electrodes placed on the forehead. The current is an alternating one of small amperage but of sufficient voltage to overcome the skin resistance. This produces an instantaneous fit. In selected cases this treatment is of great value, with a high percentage of cures, and improvement in others. Electroconvulsive therapy is of most value in involutional depression and in catatonic schizophrenia.

With the modern techniques of giving E.C.T. and with skilled nursing attention there are very few absolute contra-indications.

Preparation and Technique.—For convenience the treatment is given in the morning.

Preparation of the Patient.—This is the responsibility of the nurse in charge of the ward and includes :—

1. Consent for anæsthetic.
2. Explanation of the procedure to the patient.
3. Appropriate dressing of the patient who should not wear tight clothing or jewellery.
4. No food for 6 hours prior to anæsthetic.
5. Supervision of fluid intake during the 6-hour period.
6. Thirty minutes prior to treatment—
   a. Ask patient to pass urine.
   b. Remove dentures (if any).
   c. Reassure patient.
   d. Give premedication if ordered.
7. Observation of patient.
8. Escort patient to treatment room.

Preparation of Equipment.—Preparation of bed, trolley, oxygen, and other equipment is the responsibility of the nurse in charge of the treatment room. This should be completed and checked before the arrival of the patient.

The oxygen equipment should be placed at the head of the bed ready for instant use. The trolley will contain the following :—

Top Shelf

E.C.T. machine with electrode.

Receiver containing normal saline for the electrodes.

Wool swabs in bowl.

Gauze swabs in bowl.

Gallipot containing $\frac{1}{2}$ per cent hibitane in 70 per cent spirit.

Syringes and needles with—

   1. Sodium pentothal.
   2. Muscle relaxant, e.g., Crevidil or scoline.
   3. Atropine sulphate.

Laryngoscope.

Endotracheal tubes and lubricant, e.g., K.Y. Jelly.
Mouth gag.
Swab-holding forceps.
Bowl containing suction catheters.
Paper bag for disposal of soiled swabs.
Lower Shelf
Mackintosh and towel.
Tourniquet.
Spare oxygen face-masks in a small tray.
Spare rebreathing bags in small tray.
Spare syringes and needles in a container.
Clean air-ways and gags in a bowl.
Requirements for Resuscitation
Nikethamide.
Aminophylline.
Adrenaline 1–1000.
Ampoules of water for injection.
Intravenous infusion set.
Sodium bicarbonate 8·4 per cent solution for intravenous
  injection.
Calcium glutonate.
Lanoxin.
Methedrine.
Calcium chloride.
Vasoxine.
Hydrocortisone.
Files.
1 litre of 5 per cent dextrose.
The patient lies comfortably on his bed and whilst the
anæsthetist is injecting a muscle relaxant and pentothal intra-
venously, one of the nursing team will clean the temporal area.

The electrodes, moistened in saline, are then placed in
position on the prepared temporal site and held there by the
doctor who then, when the patient is in the ideal state of
anæsthesia, switches on the current which passes through the
brain to produce a modified epileptiform convulsion.
Occasionally respiratory difficulties follow which are combated
by administering oxygen with a pressure-bag face-mask.
Some doctors administer oxygen as a routine measure. The

patient should be observed during the post-convulsive phase, and a report made of his behaviour. These observations are very often the means of clearing up a doubtful diagnosis. Generally after an hour or two the patient is able to get up and, if he is being treated as an out-patient, to go home. There may be some memory loss for several hours, and it is desirable that he should be kept under some supervision (by a relative if he is an out-patient) for the rest of the day.

Usually between six and twelve treatments are given in a course. Some patients require periodic maintenance treatments to maintain their mental stability.

CEREBRAL SURGERY

Stereotactic Surgery.—Stereotactic surgery is now being used for treating patients with severe depression and psychoneurotic illness. Radioactive seeds which give off beta-rays are implanted immediately below the caudate nucleus and corpus striatum. Fibres concerned with emotional reaction pass through this area. These fibres can be destroyed by the radiation, but the rest of the brain is undisturbed for normal intellectual activity and normal emotional feeling.

Pre-frontal Leucotomy.—This form of treatment is very controversial and has not found favour with all psychiatrists partly because its effects are not understood, and partly because the patient may be left with an altered personality and possibly with some degree of dementia.

Pre-frontal leucotomy has been found to relieve such symptoms as excessive worry, fear, and tension which occur in many forms of mental illness such as anxiety neurosis, depression, and schizophrenia, and patients suffering from these illnesses may derive benefit from the same forms of treatment.

Pre-operative Preparation.—If the patient to be operated on is an informal patient, written authority from him and from the next of kin for the operation to be performed is necessary. For detained patients authority from one or more close relatives should be obtained.

The head is shaved, the bowels and bladder evacuated, and pre-medication given as ordered by the surgeon and anæsthetist.

The Operation.—A small hole is made in the skull on either side so that the cortex of the pre-frontal areas is exposed. A blunt instrument is introduced into the brain and is then moved upwards and downwards to divide the nerve-fibres. This is carried out on both sides, after which the wound is closed.

Post-operative Treatment.—Careful observation must be kept on the patient's general condition ; a record of the temperature, pulse, and respiration should be kept for any indication of intracranial hæmorrhage or sepsis. Careful watch should also be kept for any relapse into unconsciousness after consciousness has been regained.

Fluids can be given on gaining consciousness and light diet the day after.

A quiet darkened room is necessary to nurse the patient in, and a special watch is maintained for a few days until the doctor considers that special precautions are no longer necessary.

Confusion, apathy, or memory loss persist for varying periods after the operation, but do in most cases disappear.

CONTINUOUS NARCOSIS

Continuous narcosis is not a specific treatment in that it does not cure any particular disease, but is used to allay symptoms.

It is a treatment which is of value in cases of severe anxiety states in which there is poor emotional control, mania, and severe depression with agitation and anxiety.

Aged patients and those with organic disease are unsuitable for such treatment.

Technique.—The patient is kept in a state of sleep for the greater part of twenty-four hours a day whilst allowing him periods of wakefulness for feeding, toilet, and essential treatment.

The temperature, pulse, respiration, and blood-pressure must be recorded twice a day. The fluid intake and output must be measured and charted and the urine tested daily for albumin.

The drugs used are sodium amytal and paraldehyde, which are administered alternately.

Skill and experience will be required in adjusting the dosage of the drugs so that the timing is such that the patient is not too drowsy to be fed at meal-times, and that toxic effects are avoided.

Complications.—These are pyrexia, rise or fall in pulse-rate, fall in blood-pressure, retention of urine, raised respiratory rate, toxic confusion, chest infections.

HORMONE THERAPY

The ductless glands play a very important role in the physical and mental growth of a person. It has been noted that anyone suffering from an endocrine dysfunction has psychological symptoms as well as the usual physical disturbances. Though the use of hormonal therapy is not a regular daily feature in the care of the mentally subnormal it is used in some hospitals and it may be that more and more mentally subnormal people will receive such treatment and benefit from it in the near future.

The following conditions are encountered :—

Menopause.—Involutional melancholia and depression are the major conditions which may occur at the cessation of ovarian function. Other minor symptoms which commonly occur are headache, dizziness, and sudden repeated hot flushes. These symptoms respond readily to preparations of the hormones œstrin and stilbœstrol. The two major conditions mentioned do not respond to hormone therapy.

Impotence.—This is the inability in the male to perform or complete the sexual act. This condition has several psychological causes, most of which do not respond to hormone therapy. In some cases testosterone has been used with success. The treatment is discontinued after 14 days if no improvement is noted.

Frigidity.—This is a condition found in some women. The woman has no sexual desire and if sexual intercourse does take place she gets no sexual satisfaction from it. Small doses of either œstrin or testosterone may improve the sexual stimuli and reduce the frigidity.

Homosexuality and Excessive Sex Drive.—The force of the sexual drive in males can be reduced by treatment with the female sex hormones. With the use of these hormones some testicular atrophy may take place, though not all the sex drive is destroyed.

Male Climacteric.—The complete cessation in the production of the male sex hormone may occur in middle or later life and is indicated by symptoms of moodiness, irritability, tearfulness, and inability to concentrate.

Treatment is by testosterone by injection, 25 mg. daily until there is improvement, then methyltestosterone 5–10 mg. three times a day is given for a year.

Cretinism.—This condition is one of the classified types of primary amentia, and is caused by a lack of secretion from the thyroid gland beginning in fœtal life. Treatment is by thyroid extract given as soon as the condition is diagnosed.

Thyrotoxicosis.—Over-activity of the thyroid gland. It is thought by some authorities that thyrotoxicosis is caused by the emotional mechanism acting upon the endocrine system.

In cases requiring thyroidectomy, the operation may be followed by a degree of myxœdema and may require treatment with thyroid hormone.

Myxœdema.—Under-activity of the thyroid gland. This condition produces mental changes such as sluggishness, apathy, melancholia, or mania, and the speech is slow and mumbling. The treatment is with thyroid hormone, the administration of which will require care as it may accentuate confusion and delirium, and precipitate death.

Addison's Disease.—This condition is associated with under-activity of the adrenal glands. The symptoms of the disease may include such psychiatric states as apathy, negativism, depression, and irritability.

In the treatment of this condition beneficial results may be obtainable from the use of cortisone, an extract from the adrenal gland.

Study is still going on into the relationship between endocrine dysfunction and psychiatric diseases.

PSYCHOTHERAPY AND COUNSELLING

Psychotherapy is a form of mental therapy which involves the establishing of a positive relationship between therapist and patient. It is only suitable for patients who are able to freely associate. It seeks to explore and modify the patient's behaviour problems and relationship difficulties, some of which may be acknowledged by the patient though he probably does not understand them.

Counselling is most frequently directed towards the solution of specific problems of adaptation as they occur from day to day, and it aims at finding a practical solution without attempting to change the basic personality.

In young children psychotherapy aims at providing the warmth and affection of which the child has been starved. This applies in particular to young and older children who come from severely disturbed backgrounds and have become confused in their emotional relationships, resulting in an anxious, isolated withdrawnness over their own apparent disloyalties towards the parents, and their parents' disloyalties towards them. Therapy with these children takes place on an emotional plane, the therapist providing a father- and mother-substitute. Very often it is necessary for the therapist to resort to hugging and cuddling in order to transfer the sense of security of a relationship to the child. Once this has been achieved social adjustment will follow.

Emotional problems will result in the patient appearing to be lower grade than he really is, because his functioning level is being disturbed. Therefore the criterion for withholding psychotherapy treatment should not be the patient's intelligence quotient, otherwise he may be deprived of treatment which might be successful in restoring effective mental functioning.

The aims of psychotherapy are :—

1. To reduce suspiciousness felt towards outsiders.
2. To release aggression.
3. To encourage feelings of self-confidence and self-work.
4. To develop a sense of responsibility for actions.

Treatment should begin from the moment of admission and should not be left to the patient to make excuses for his admission. A discussion of the events leading to the patient's admission, his prospects, the rules of the hospital, and the privileges he can gain, will help to overcome uncertainty and hostility. The therapist's ready offer to mediate between the hospital and the patient to shorten the stay in hospital as much as possible, coming at this difficult moment, will help to initiate the warm and supportive relationship required by the therapist.

The therapist's mediation should lead to an acceptance by the patient of his group relationships and to a realization that the community at large expects him to fit in with its requirements. He must be made to realize that he is neither clever enough nor strong enough to set himself up against society, and that he will get hurt unless he co-operates with society. Many frictions between himself and society are due to misunderstandings and to his desire to hide his ignorance.

The community requires him, like everyone else, to accept a reasonable amount of frustration and to exercise control over his emotional life. Psychotherapy does not aim to cure mental subnormality nor to make him function to his full mental capacity, though it does introduce and make acceptable new behaviour patterns.

The environment in which the patient lives can effect the outcome of psychotherapy. It is essential that, as well as providing shelter where the patient can be calm or deterred by the fear of long hospitalization, it should be more positive in providing a community life which is understood and accepted as a preparatory stage for living and working in the community outside. The staff–patient relationship should be right, and opportunities should be given to the patient to demonstrate his improved social competence. One of the difficulties facing the nurse and the therapist is the indefinite nature of his stay in hospital. The patient realizes that, had he been committed to prison, it would have been for a specified sentence. All this creates an atmosphere of distrust, fear, apprehension, and insecurity. Only by breaking down the repressive impersonal atmosphere of the ward, by making every patient feel his importance and trustworthiness, and his individuality, can the nurse and therapist penetrate the protective armour the patient has surrounded himself with.

CHAPTER XVIII

PSYCHOLOGICAL DEVELOPMENT

INTRODUCTORY

In the General Nursing Council's syllabus for the Certificate of Mental Subnormality Nursing, emphasis has been placed upon the development and activities of the human being whose mental and physical characteristics blend to form a whole.

In order that the nurse may recognize and observe the unusual behaviour of her patients and understand why their pattern of behaviour is such, she must first appreciate what constitutes normal behaviour and development.

It is important that the nurse to the mentally subnormal child should have an understanding of a normal child's psychological needs, and realize that the same needs are experienced by her patients and play the same important part in their psychological development. Their need of a mother's love, of affection, and of security are just as great.

The social surroundings, the environment, and the people in it all influence the individual person's behaviour.

During the further consideration of elementary psychology the study of the mental mechanisms is included to illustrate how the human mind has developed means of overcoming and forgetting unpleasant and painful emotions and disturbing memories. Normal people exhibit these traits, but when they become a means of escaping from one's problems, and a method of self-deception, abnormal behaviour results.

The normal workings of these mechanisms can be observed in the mentally subnormal person as well as the mechanisms of escape and self-deception.

The mind and the body are interdependent, the well-being of the one being dependent upon the other and vice versa. As will be explained in Chapter XXV, any emotional disturbance upsets the normal physiological processes, often with severe consequences ; for example, the person suffering from jaundice loses interest in life and may seek the opportunity to commit suicide, but on recovery from the disease regains his interest in life once more.

The following sections explain the various factors and processes which contribute to the development of a normal personality.

THE MOTHER-FATHER RELATIONSHIP

The mother-father relationship should be a stable and lasting association. It existed before the child arrived and will continue long after the child has grown up and left home. It is important, therefore, that the child does not interfere with this relationship. Father should always remain just that bit more important to Mother than the child is.

The father should show his love for the mother so that she feels secure in their love for each other and is thus free to devote her time to the child without being anxious about her husband's love. Any anxiety experienced by the mother is invariably transferred to the child, who will become affected by her disturbed mind.

Parents should never feel that they are pathologically responsible for their child being difficult or abnormal, as there are factors which play an even greater part in the development of emotional instability in a child, as for example :—

1. The total environment from the time of conception.
2. Physical health.
3. Temperament.
4. Unstable central nervous system.

The age limits set out in the following pages are purely for guidance. Some children attain a 7-year-old child's standard of efficiency at 5 years of age, and another child may not achieve such a standard until he has reached the age of 9, but will still be normal mentally.

No hard-and-fast rules can be laid down concerning the age at which a child can reach the various milestones of development ; all children differ in their physical and mental abilities.

MOTHER AND CHILD

Human behaviour begins developing with life, and it grows from complete dependence to almost complete independence in adult life.

It is the experiences occurring during the first years of life that are of lasting importance. Psychologists agree that the development of a healthy, mature, and stable person depends primarily on the mother–child relationship. Indeed, the original principles of the Freudian psychoanalysis were to help people to bring back to consciousness the feelings and memories of their past life to help them to gain an insight into their adult relationship difficulties.

Everything that happens to a child during the early months of life is related to the satisfying of his primitive physical needs, such as food, warmth, and comfort.

When a baby is in his mother's arms and feeding from her breast, he feels contented, happy, and secure. At first he only regards her as a source of food and it is not until a little later that she becomes recognized as a separate person.

Breast-feeding is an intimate function for both mother and child, and it is on this emotionally satisfying relationship that true foundations of stable development are laid.

The child's first experiences of satisfaction are when being fed and feeling warm and comfortable. Feeding is the most important experience and if it is carried out in an unsatisfactory manner it will assist the development of emotional instability.

Serious reasons for unsatisfactory feeding may be :—

1. The mother did not want the baby and therefore it is a nuisance which has to be tolerated. The child is fed at irregular intervals and only at the convenience of the mother.

2. Low mentality of the mother who without constant supervision is incapable of feeding the child properly.

3. More commonly the mother is unhappy, which is due to three main reasons :—

a. People have made the mother anxious. They have criticized her ways of handling the baby, and suggested that the progress of the child is not satisfactory. This criticism tends to make the mother anxious and cause her to lose her confidence in handling the baby.

b. If the marriage is unhappy the mother will feel insecure and will transfer that feeling to the child.

c. If the mother has too much work to do, and cannot cope with it, no matter how much she loves her child she cannot avoid the feelings of anxiety, frustration, and defeat. These are feelings that the child quickly becomes sensitive to in his relationship with his mother.

Through this intimate relationship, his emotions of love and anger develop and the intensity of these only becomes modified by experience. Memories of what has happened before help the child to control his feelings.

His confidence in his mother can be greatly improved if his daily routine is regular and constant.

Weaning is a critical period in the life of the child and should be carried out gradually. He should be allowed to adjust himself to the change step by step. Other situations which provide ample opportunity for the experience of love between child and mother, such as bathing and toilet, should receive greater attention.

When the child is weaned the chances of conflict with authority, represented in the parents, are ever present and the anxious parents will do battle with the child over simple and foolish things, often because of poor advice given to them by neighbours and friends. As an example, the child may one day decide that he doesn't want to eat his dinner, but the anxious parent feels that he must eat and insists on him doing so. This produces a battle of wills and once the child has experienced this clash he will use it as a means of 'getting at' his parents every time he feels annoyed. The best advice that can be given to these parents is that, once the child has refused to eat, not to get involved with him. If he doesn't eat his dinner he will be ready for his tea, and he will realize that his behaviour is affecting himself more than anyone else and will quickly stop misbehaving.

With the child's development his dependence upon his mother for other satisfactions increases.

Towards the end of the first year of life, this sense of security and confidence is still centred round his mother and he quickly becomes insecure and frustrated if he is separated from her for long.

At the age of 2 he may relive his earlier emotional life and make demands upon his mother similar to those he made while only a small baby.

The mother–child relationship is generally smooth and satisfactory to both at the age of 3, the child treating his mother as a favoured companion and becoming less demanding towards her.

Mother's authority becomes a thing to resist at 3–4 years of age, and usually only for the sake of resisting. Fortunately for the mother's peace of mind, by the time the child has reached the age of 5 he is again happy in his obedience to her authority and Mother is once again the centre of his world and he needs her affection just as much as ever.

Behaviour changes in the young child tend to be patterned and predictable and the relationship between the mother and child depends entirely on how skilfully the child is treated.

FATHER–CHILD RELATIONSHIP

To the consternation of many fathers, young pre-school children tend to constantly rebuff their efforts of help and demand that Mother does it for them. If the child wakes up during the night it is Mother who is called for to give comfort and reassurance, not Father.

Once the hazards of the early years are past, the father–child relationship develops into a smoother association than that between the mother and child. This may be because the child's feelings about his father are not so tense and sensitive as they are about his mother.

At the age of 4, the rebellious streak in the child may be changed into obedience by a word from Father who is not only a respected disciplinarian, but an authority who can be quoted outside.

Though the child is still fond and proud of his father at the age of 5 it is still Mother who is the centre of his world.

At the age of 6 the child struggles to overthrow the authoritative power of the mother and may become defiant and violent towards her, but his relationship with his father is at its best and he has more respect for his father's authority than for that of his mother.

In most families there is a need for Father to stabilize things when the child is 6, but these needs become less intense, until at the age of 8 the need for a mother's love overshadows any other relationship and Father as a result feels left out. The child may also become jealous of his father's show of affection towards his mother.

At the age of 9 new friends are made outside the immediate family circle and as a result the child is less demanding to either his mother or father. He does, however, accept what the parents of his friends say as being of greater importance than what his own parents say.

Father's technical knowledge and ability become increasingly respected and the 9-year-old child begins to share an interest with Father and the things they do together.

Ten is the most successful age in the father–child relationship. It is an age when Father is idolized by his child, who likes to be alone with him and to share things with him.

Unfortunately for Father this phase does not last, but other phases come to take its place.

THE SCHOOL-AGE CHILD

The first school experience for some children occurs rather early in life. Many start nursery school as early as 3 or 4 years of age, but for the majority of children this big event in their lives does not take place until they have reached the age of 5.

Providing the development of the child has been normal he will be active and full of energy, and though he will be far from his maximum muscular control and co-ordination he will have sufficient skills to make use of the abundant opportunities for movement and activity.

A 5-year-old child uses his mental activities as much as he uses his physical capabilities. His environment is constantly stimulating his thought-processes and he is constantly being urged on to investigate things for himself. His power of speech is a great help to him, its power being in his ability to ask questions about anything that puzzles him.

When a child enters school for the first time, he is overawed at the strangeness of the building, at meeting for the first time large groups of children who are strangers to him, and at having to attach himself to a strange adult whose ways he does not know or understand.

On entering school he has left behind for the first time the sheltered environment of home and the security and confidence of the presence of Mother.

Big demands are made on the child's ability to adjust himself. The ease with which he adapts himself to his new way of life depends upon the soundness of his earlier emotional development and his sense of security within the family circle. A child with a sound background makes a reasonably easy adjustment and presents very few problems.

At first the child's play is individualistic, even though he may be playing within a group. If, for instance, he were playing football and the ball were passed to him, he would keep it to himself and lose it in trying to score goals, rather than pass it on to someone else who might be in a better position to score.

The infant schoolchild's play is imaginative and make-believe, often having very little relationship to his real experiences and being quite different from reality.

Think for a moment of the number of small children you know who call themselves 'Bill' and 'Tom' or some such name during their fantasy play. The child will often dress himself up to fit the part he is acting. Any figurehead known and admired by him will be made use of to build his play around.

Very gradually during his early school life, the child will devote less and less time to fantasy play, but imaginative and make-believe play becomes more related to reality, taking the form of dramatizing and acting. Doctors, and Mothers and Fathers, and Cowboys and Indians dominate his play.

Around the age of 7 he is able to co-operate with other children in play without being too aware of himself and too domineering.

At this age-level his need of the supporting presence of an adult and the emotional satisfaction of his relationships with Father and Mother become less.

This is one of the most stable periods of his childhood, but will be followed by the ferment of adolescence.

By the time the child reaches 7–10 years of age he begins to enjoy school and is unhappy over enforced absence. He has acquired an enthusiasm for school and an interest in all the other children attending. His world is steadily widening and more people and interests are entering it.

Although by this time he becomes more completely independent of grown-ups, he still needs the sustaining power of security within the group. This he will find within the groups which children of this age form, such as gangs and secret societies from which adults are excluded.

In the child's progress through the various school levels he gradually begins to welcome opportunities for learning ; he pursues knowledge, which leads to a considerable increase in manipulative skills and in the use and understanding of language.

All normal healthy schoolchildren are interested in their physical activities, and all the time they are actively engaged they shout, sing, and talk unceasingly.

It is only through exercising their bodies and extending their experiences in many directions that they can develop their skills and sensitivity, and understanding of the world in which they live. The best way for any child to learn is through his own experiences.

As he grows older he prefers to work and play in a group where he can identify himself with his team even at the cost of his own desires.

At about 10 or 11 years of age he begins to show hostility towards grown-ups and authority, but he enjoys belonging to the Scouts and club movements, even though he will be subjected to their disciplinary code.

Collecting stamps, car numbers, and train numbers plays a prominent part in his life to the extent of competition, rivalry, bargaining, and ' swopping '.

Up to this age children of both sexes mix quite happily, but look upon each other with scorn and would rather die than be seen playing with each other.

During the later years of childhood closer and more lasting friendships are formed outside the family circle, which makes a stage of further development towards emotional maturity.

16

The schoolchild is a practical person. He is interested in real and concrete things. Even in hospital, where he is deprived of the normal environment and relationships, his interests and quest for knowledge should be satisfied by sensible answers to questions and a reasonable explanation given at a simple level which he can grasp.

The child who has had the opportunity to live a full and normal childhood in every way is best equipped for the changes and adjustments required of him in adolescence.

ADOLESCENCE

Adolescence represents the final stage of development towards adulthood. This stage varies with different people, but it covers roughly the period between the ages of 12 and 18 years.

It can be divided into two distinct phases :—

1. **Stage of Puberty.**—Physical changes towards adulthood take place. All the secondary sexual characteristics begin to appear, such as deepening of the voice and the growth of hair on the face in the male. At the same time as physical growth and sexual maturity are taking place, the period of adolescence is the time when the child achieves the final stage in his growth towards emotional independence of his parents.

During the stage of puberty psychological changes take place. Swings in moods and attitudes are constantly occurring. The child once more passes through a period of introspection ; he retreats into solitariness and a life of fantasy and day-dreaming.

The adolescent is whole-heartedly defiant of authority and is argumentative and boastful. He enjoys his emotions and his feelings of revolt towards those in authority.

In his world of day-dreaming he delights in self-sacrifice and enjoys watching himself objectively, when he may contemplate suicide ; fortunately he is rarely serious ; therefore there is no danger in these feeling-states. All adolescents have a period during their daily lives when they are going to capture the world.

2. **Stage of Maturity.**—In the later period of adolescence when the adolescent is approaching adulthood, he has been

able to adjust himself emotionally to the extensive physical changes that have taken place.

The stresses and turbulence of the puberty stage have been adjusted and most conflicts resolved. Not until all the over-whelming forces have been adequately dealt with has maturity been reached.

The Adolescent in Difficulties.—Most of the difficulties are associated with the lack of some of the fundamental needs, such as security and affection, the need for independence, and a change of interest.

Financial security within the home and in the job ; affection and understanding from parents and friends ; the need for independence and release from the parents' authority ; and a satisfaction for the craving for adventure, are all important and essential psychological needs, which if not satisfied may produce instability.

ADULTHOOD

Once adulthood has been reached it does not indicate the finality of development, either mentally or physically, but it should be a stage where a person is capable of accepting responsibility, of acting on his own initiative, and of managing his own personal relations with other people. The adult should be able to live in harmony within the community. To do this he must be able to control his impulses and desires.

Adulthood can be divided into three phases : (1) The young adult ; (2) the period of middle age ; (3) the period of old age.

The Young Adult.—This period should be exhilarating—the person is at the peak of his physical power ; for the majority matrimony and parenthood lie ahead and all the joys of a happy family life.

The responses made by the adult will have been pre-determined by the pattern of his psychological development from early life. Those adults with an inadequate background are unable to accept a subordinate status if in the past they have always been in the limelight. They have difficulty in adjusting themselves to a new discipline. This type of person is unable to settle down in one job and is constantly moving from one to another.

Starting a family makes fresh demands on the emotional life of the parents, on the father in particular, who, while he feels he is being neglected by his wife, has heavier responsibilities to carry with the advent of a new offspring.

The Period of Middle Age.—The need for a middle-aged person to adjust himself to a change of circumstances arises out of his declining physical abilities. For the athlete, the decline takes place early and he has to be content with the less strenuous activities.

Intellectual development comes to an end, but a more mature judgement on problems is possible due to the wide range of experiences gained in earlier life.

The middle-aged person has his problems ; he is slower at assimilating new ideas and has greater difficulty in recalling past experiences.

The physical changes that take place are more dramatic in a woman than in a man. At the age of puberty they both achieve the child-bearing potentials, but it is only in the middle-aged woman that these potentials cease to function at the menopause. The sense of loss is inevitable ; to the woman the child-bearing age is the most important period of her life and it demands great powers of adjustment for her to reconcile herself to this loss.

In the middle-aged man there is only a diminished virility, and because of his varied interests he is able to adjust himself more easily.

The ideal way of accepting the progress of time is never to dwell with the past and to accept the challenges of new experiences.

The Period of Old Age.—Some old people have difficulty in being able to face up to reality and of accepting their age. They will not accept the progressive decline in their mental and physical capabilities. Memory declines ; to recall fairly recent experiences is difficult, but those experiences which took place in youth can be recalled most vividly. Deterioration of the senses of hearing and vision also takes place and in extreme cases will create in the aged person a feeling of isolation.

To adjust himself to the approach of old age a person must be prepared to accept the fact that it does have its effect on both the physical and intellectual sphere to such an extent that it will impose severe limitations. He must be prepared to compromise with his old age and take up new interests which are within his capabilities without being too strenuous. In accepting the limitations it will be possible to live well a full life within himself.

Old people who are unable to adjust themselves successfully, and who allow their interests to go without replacing them, quickly become isolated from the rest of the community, and because of a lack of stimulation become once more introverted, and rapidly develop mental decay—a pathetic picture of what could have been a useful life being allowed to wither away.

CHAPTER XIX

PATTERNS OF BEHAVIOUR

Aims and Methods of Psychology.—Psychology is the study of the normal mind, and by a series of methods it attempts to study how a person behaves in his environment.

In any environment there is a standard considered as normal, but this will differ between societies. For example, in England it is the law and custom for a man to have but one wife, while a Moslem is permitted to have more than one. These different patterns are described as the cultural patterns of a society.

One method of studying behaviour is by questioning the person, but there is a distinct disadvantage, as the patient does not always answer truthfully.

Other methods of studying behaviour are :—

1. *Introspection.*—A science of self-criticism (self-examination), asking oneself " Why do I behave in such a way ?"

2. *Observation.*—Watching and studying the other person's behaviour in his environment.

3. *Experimental Psychology.*—Experimenting on a person to find out why his pattern of behaviour changes under certain conditions. The examiner is in a normal environment throughout the experiment, which must be uniform.

Comparison.—Much light is thrown on to man's mental processes by comparing them with those observed in other members of the animal kingdom. Comparisons are made of the behaviour of the primitive races with that of the civilized races of mankind ; and the mental processes of the child in its various stages of growth and development with those of the adult.

Comparisons are made of the mind in health and the mind which is defective or disordered.

Tropism.—This is an unlearnt form of behaviour or response, which is not under the control of a nervous system. It is the simplest form of adaptive pattern reaction which results from a chemical or physical stimulus. Such reactions are to be found in plants whose roots grow downwards—positive geotropism—and stems upwards towards the light—heliotropism.

Reflex Action.—This is the lowest form of behaviour in man. It differs from tropism in the fact that it is the response of an impulse conducted along a nerve-fibre. Reflex action requires :—

1. A sensory end-organ.
2. A sensory neuron.
3. A connector neuron.
4. A motor neuron.
5. A motor end-organ.

These structures activated in the simple reflex are called the reflex arc. The action is a uniform one which is not necessarily under the control of the will, its value being in the protection of the person against serious injury. The will can enter into the act and can control the reflex, when it becomes known as an inhibited reflex.

Conditioned Reflex.—A conditioned response or a conditioned behaviour is a form of behaviour which is apparently learnt, but which is dependent upon a set of fixed conditions. For example, Pavlov experimented on dogs ; when taking food to the dogs he rang a bell, until the food and the ringing of a bell were associated ; then later he rang the bell but provided no food, but the dogs still salivated as much as when the food was served.

Automatic Action.—This consists of an acquired series of movements which, owing to repetition, have lost all need of conscious attention ; there is an absence of any movement idea. Walking, for example, is an automatic action and does not, in fact, require any thought.

Habit.—A form of behaviour which is dependent upon certain conditions and is very closely bound up with conditioned reflex. It is a stereotyped form of behaviour which requires very little conscious thought and produces neither a feeling of strain nor of effort. Behind a habit is the driving force of a motive, and the chief troubles in many of the mentally subnormals' dirty and destructive habits can often be attributed to certain motives. The treatment consists first of all in helping the patient to break the undesirable habit by removing him from the situation which provokes the motives, and secondly, by encouraging the formation of new habits connected to some other motive which is strong enough to ensure its permanency.

Motivation.—A motive is a tendency to activity started by a persistent stimulus or drive and ended by an adjustment.

An instinct is an impulse or drive to follow, without training, a certain pattern of behaviour, which is common to members of the same species. Nowadays the use of the term ' instinct ' is usually limited to the field of animal behaviour.

The insect's instinctive behaviour fits it for a certain form of life which has as its basis the preservation and perpetuation of the species.

In man, behaviour is not stereotyped. His behaviour is influenced by learning and by cultural factors. The behaviour response of two people to the same type of motive may be completely different. The behaviour pattern is concerned with bodily needs, and with dealing with the environment, i.e., the motives are not active all the time ; they become active when stirred up by some situation.

Some of these motives are :—

1. Parental motive.
2. Sex motive.
3. Combat or pugnacious motive.
4. Gregarious motive.
5. Acquisitive motive.

1. *Parental Motive.*—This is a drive or force in behaviour which makes a person adopt a mother-like attitude towards others, usually those with an inferior physique.

The normal standards are those accepted in that person's cultural pattern ; the standards set by the cultural and social pattern vary in different countries.

2. *Sex Motive.*—This is a drive or force which has been modified in our country. It is a great driving force which

makes a person seek out another person of the opposite sex with the purpose of procreating children. Society exercises a certain code of behaviour on the person exercising this energy ; it demands that the man provides a home and that he marries the woman of his choice and works to maintain her and his children.

Again, the cultural pattern modifies the sex motive and so determines what is normal in the expression of the sex motive.

Margaret Mead, a widely travelled lady, during one of her travels abroad came across three islands which were in close proximity to each other, but on each island the cultural-pattern control over the sexual motive urge was different. For example :—

a. Arapesh : The men and women are gentle people who look after their children and love each other. Theirs is a non-aggressive cultural pattern.

b. Mundugumor : The man and woman are aggressive towards each other and severely attack each other. They have children, but they do not treat them kindly. At feeding time food is forced down the child's throat which often chokes it. Many of the children die from choking.

Here is a social pattern of no desire to have children, and of aggressive sex behaviour.

c. Tchambali : The male members dress themselves up in fancy clothes and play that part played by the female in our own society. The woman adopts the masculine role.

3. *The Pugnacious or Aggressive Motive.*—The drive or force which gives us a desire to harm something or somebody in our environment. Adler said that his view was that this stems from the fact that as children we naturally feel weak in relation to the outside world and inferior to those around us. We never completely lose this feeling of inferiority, as a result of which we strive hard to prove to people how superior we are.

Some people set themselves ambitions which are far out of their reach and then suddenly, after a few failures, realize that they cannot rise to such heights, and because of this they worry, develop a great sense of inferiority, and become neurotic, unless they set themselves another target which is well within their reach. This is termed 're-adjustment.'

The adolescents who attire themselves in modern dress may quite well be compensating for their inferiority. They are identifying themselves as belonging to a well-known gang.

The bully in the ward may be the inferior type of person trying to attract attention to himself. His aggression may be overcome if his energies can be re-directed. Praise for work done and encouragement given to aim at greater success in some job may succeed where criticism and punishment fail.

The psychologist Freud said that people who were aggressive in any way were deriving pleasure out of their aggression, and he believed that anything we did originated from the sex motive, which shows itself as two different complexes, one typical of the male—the Œdipus complex—and the other typical of the female—the Electra complex.

The Œdipus complex : In early life the young male child is much more dependent upon his mother than his father, and because of his intimate contact with her, he falls in love with her, and in his extreme love and affection he rivals his father for her love. As a result a hate for his father enters his life. Realizing that there will be many advantages in showing a liking for him, the feeling of hate is repressed (shut down in the back of the mind) and in its place an apparent approval is shown.

The Electra complex : The female child hates and rivals the mother for the love of the father.

4. *Gregarious Motive.*—People usually go around in herds or groups and society looks upon the ' lone wolf ' as being abnormal. Most of us require the comfort of other peoples' presence. There is also security in the company of others. Take, for instance, the man in the midst of a football crowd. He will array himself in the colours of his team and behave foolishly, yet away from the crowd his behaviour changes as he loses the security of the mass of people.

Patients alone and in a corner doing nothing feel insecure. The nurse should encourage them to join others in their activities so that they will get the feeling of security of companionship.

5. *Acquisitive or Hoarding Motive.*—Squirrels hoard nuts, schoolboys collect stamps, marbles, etc. There is a drive or urge to collect things ; the value of them does not matter. A

patient, for instance, who carries around with him a bag full of what we would consider to be rubbish, probably does it for prestige and probably derives pleasure out of it, and the admiration of the other patients. Efforts should be made to direct that energy into other more sociable channels, such as collecting silver paper and firewood.

CHAPTER XX

INTELLIGENCE AND INTELLIGENCE TESTING

INTELLIGENCE, like electricity, is easier to talk about than it is to define. The psychiatrist uses the word to mean 'the power to think abstractly' and the teacher uses it to mean 'the power to acquire knowledge'. For the nurse the definition 'the ability to reason things out' will be adequate.

Intelligence is a factor which varies in individuals, even in close blood relations. It alters at different ages, and at 14–16 years of age it levels out. Most authorities assume that mental growth ends between the ages of 14 and 16 years. After the age of 21 years a gradual deterioration begins to take place, which increases after the age of 72 years. In some people rapid deterioration takes place much earlier in life.

The growth of intelligence can be affected by many factors, such as accidents involving the brain, illness, poor and inadequate nutrition, lack of suitable opportunities on which the mind can feed, and the lack of satisfaction of the emotional needs in early childhood. Even if all the ideal conditions prevail for mental growth to take place, unless there is present the inherited or inborn potential for normal development, the potential maximum cannot be increased.

It is the inherited potential which is assessed by means of intelligence tests. These intelligence tests are so devised to offset as far as possible any previous learning or opportunities, and to measure not what the person has learnt, but his capacity to learn.

All intelligence tests are first of all standardized before being used to assess a person's intelligence; that is, when a test has been devised it is applied to a large number of people of one age-group and from all walks of life. From the findings of the scores achieved by those tested an average mark can be calculated for that age. By this means tests and average marks for each age-level are devised and calculated so that a table of normal marks can be prepared for each age-group.

The score of many intelligence tests is expressed as the mental age in order to make comparisons of people of different ages. The mental score is expressed as the intelligence quotient, which is based on the relationship of the calendar age (chronological age) and the mental age, multiplied by 100 to give the percentile.

The intelligence quotient is

$$\frac{\text{Mental age (test age)}}{\text{Calendar age (chronological age)}} \times 100 = \text{I.Q.}$$

For example, if a child has a mental age of 7 years and a calendar age of 14 years his intelligence quotient and percentile would be

$$\frac{\text{Mental age } 7}{\text{Calendar age } 14} \times 100 = \text{I.Q. } 50$$

The intelligence quotient of most people falls roughly between 90 and 110 ; this is termed 'average'. The number of

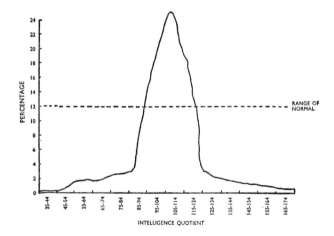

people whose intelligence quotient deviates from the average becomes less the farther away from the average one gets. For every one person there is on the below-average side, a corresponding one appears on the above-average side. The I.Q. distribution curve appears roughly as illustrated above.

Behaviour difficulties will arise with children whose intelligence quotient is on either side of the average curve unless their individual needs are understood and met at the level of their intellectual ability.

The graph shows that half the population has an average intelligence quotient, a quarter is below the average and a quarter above the average.

Intelligence tests, though widely used, are still subject to doubt and criticism, particularly from the legal and educational professions. These tests are used to test the mentally subnormal patient, to assess his degree of mental ability, but are not used as a criterion for the diagnosis of mental subnormality. There is, however, some relationship between the I.Q. and the degree of mental subnormality; for instance, an I.Q. of under 75 is subnormal and 75 to 90 is borderline.

INTELLIGENCE TESTS

It is essential that the tester be patient and that he take his time over applying the tests.

Before beginning the test, time must be taken to put the patient's mind at rest and to gain his confidence and co-operation. Nervousness and fatigue will have an important influence over the results of the tests.

The patient's attitude, his approach to the tests, and the way he attacks the problems will give important information on his mental capacity.

Mental tests may be divided into the following four groups :—

1. Tests of scholastic attainment.
2. Tests of range of general or common-sense knowledge.
3. Serial 'intelligence' tests, standardized to age.
4. Tests of special mental factors and specific abilities.

   1. Tests of Scholastic Attainment.—Scholastic ability and social ability are not identical, but they are frequently associated and a defect in one usually means a defect in the other.

In the case of children attending school, reports of attainment, rate of progress, and educability can be obtained from the school-teacher. In the case of adolescents and adults, where no school report is available, they are given passages to read from selected books and asked to explain the meaning of what they have read, to write sentences from dictation, and to do mentally and on paper simple sums in arithmetic and problems in money change. The aim of these tests is to find out if the person has sufficient scholastic knowledge to manage his affairs in a reasonably efficient manner.

2. Tests of Common-sense Knowledge.—The normal person has an innate ability to acquire knowledge of things around him and soon becomes acquainted with their names and their uses.

A mentally subnormal person is different; he lacks the power of initiative, observation, attention, memory, discrimination, and reasoning; he therefore misses most of the environmental stimuli.

The best means of estimating a person's general knowledge is by a questionnaire arranged so that it tests his knowledge and understanding of things and events which are a part of his normal life. The questions can be so arranged as to be suitable for all ages.

3. Graded Serial Tests.—The most commonly used test of this kind is the Stanford-Binet test which is a revised version of the original Binet and Simon test.

There are tests for each year of life from 2–14 ; a test for the average adult, and 3 tests for superior adults.

For the ages from 2–5 years there are tests for each 6 months, and in each 6-monthly test there are 6 sub-tests, each one to represent monthly development. For children from 6–14 years each 12-monthly period has 6 sub-tests, each one corresponding to a 2-monthly stage of development.

To begin testing, the person is given tests corresponding to two years below his calendar age and increased until no results are obtained. For each year's test completed he is credited with the mental age of the highest age test completed, and is also credited with an additional one month mental age for each sub-test completed between 2 and 5 years, and an additional two months for each sub-test between 6 and 14 years where he has failed to pass the complete test of that year.

4. Tests of Special Mental Factors and Specific Abilities.

—Most of these tests are performance tests and have been devised to gauge the special mental factors and specific abilities of the person to be tested, such as memory, perception, association, relationships, reasoning, prevision, planning, constructiveness, and social sense.

The tests commonly in use to ascertain these special attributes are :—

a. Wechsler Intelligence Tests.—The Wechsler test is a battery of ten tests, each one being devised to test one or more of the special attributes, as follows :—

Information test : This test will assess the person's intellectual ability, the test result depending upon the educational and cultural opportunities available to the individual.

Comprehension test : A person's common sense and personality are ascertained with this test.

Arithmetical reasoning test : The result is influenced by the person's education and occupation. Fluctuations in attention and emotion will also affect the results.

Memory span of digits : This is a good test of retentiveness.

Similarities test : This test provides a good indication of the person's logical thinking processes.

Picture arrangement test : This test is useful in summing up the ability to comprehend and to size up a total situation.

Picture completion test : This tests the ability to distinguish essential from inessential details.

Block design : This test assesses the ability to recognize and reproduce designs, and tests the general intellectual ability.

Digit symbol test : A test useful to assess the subject's perceptual ability.

Object assembly test : By asking the person to put together three sets of pieces to form three different objects, his perceptual ability is tested.

b. Porteous Maze.—A series of mazes increasing in difficulty, devised to test the prevision and planning ability of a person.

c. Raven Matrices Test.—This is a perceptual test of intelligence. The person has to select the correct pattern from a number of alternatives to complete the design.

d. Vineland Social Scale.—This test attempts to assess the mentally subnormal's social sense and social competency.

e. Rorschach Ink-blot Personality Test.—A series of twenty standard ink-blots ; the patient has to say in turn what each one suggests to him.   This test assesses the creative imagination and also gives information on fundamental personality traits.

CHAPTER XXI

LEARNING, REMEMBERING, AND FORGETTING

LEARNING

A DEFINITION of learning is ' the modification and control of behaviour so as to make it more effective and better adapted to the situation present '.

Learning is obviously dependent upon the sensory processes, such as seeing and hearing, for it comes from responding to their stimulations. It is known, however, that people born blind and deaf do learn motor skills. Nevertheless, there is usually a decrease in the progress of learning with a decrease in sensory stimulation.

Before learning can take place a certain stage of development of the body is necessary. Intelligence is also necessary for learning. If a subject is not understood it cannot be learnt.

Conditions of Learning.—

1. *Repetition.*—A person usually needs to repeat the learning situation. This is not always necessary, as learning is occasionally resultant from incidental observation, imitation, and as a result of a single emotional experience (if a child burns his hand he will in future avoid the pain-producing stimulus).

Without the driving force of a motive behind the learning situation, learning may not take place or it may be difficult. The importance of repetition lies in the fact that it involves repeating other conditions which facilitate learning.

2. *Effect.*—The responses made to a situation which appealed to and satisfied a person tend to be retained in the memory whilst those which fail to satisfy are rejected.

3. *Intensity of Motive.*—If a teacher in the course of one of his lectures makes the remark : " You will be asked something about this in your examination ", the student will learn all the facts of that one subject. Rivalry will stimulate great effort

to learn, all outside stimuli being overshadowed by the desire to learn. Often the student with the most to lose if he fails in the examination will put the most effort into his study. A patient motivated by the prospect of increased rewards will tend to respond quicker to the training he is receiving.

4. *Recency.*—Recent experiences are as a rule more vivid than earlier ones, but on occasion the person's emotional mechanism may affect his behaviour to such an extent that he fails to register any of the experiences that have taken place recently.

5. *Primacy.*—First experiences have a long-lasting effect upon the memory. Novelty of first experiences has a great tendency to attract attention and therefore assist in learning.

Types of Learning.—

1. *By Acquiring Skills.*—Through utilizing our physical and mental abilities we learn ways of accomplishing tasks through exercise and repetition, individual technique being adjusted in the light of experience.

2. *By Learning Facts.*—The learner has to depend upon facts which he acquires from his daily contacts and experience. These facts may be right or wrong.

3. *By Learning to acquire certain Attitudes of Mind.*—The way a person feels for his subject or work, etc., is developed in such a way as to give him the desire to learn. The pain–pleasure principle will influence the development of feeling, the greater the reward—which could be promotion prospects for becoming proficient in the activity—the stronger the feeling-tone, resulting in greater learning.

Ways of Learning.—

1. *Trial and Error.*—This is wasteful in time and money, and is an unintelligent but very effective way of learning. This is a system of learning adopted by animals. Human beings also make free use of it.

2. *Learning by Insight and Observation.*—Some investigators into the mechanism of learning emphasize the fact that learning by trial and error precedes learning by insight. Intelligence and the power of thought are essential for learning by insight and observation. This method demands that the learner stop to observe and to think in order that he may ascertain the best way of carrying out the task ahead.

3. *Learning by Response Conditioning.*—A new reaction to a situation is developed by the response to an added stimulus which is powerful enough to make the change desirable. Through the appeal of persuasion and the stimulus of rewards the misbehaving patient is encouraged to learn a more acceptable behaviour. As in trial and error, new skills are learnt by rejecting inadequate methods until the correct method has been found.

4. *Play for Children.*—Play is necessary for the development of the child, and time and opportunity for play should be allowed in every daily time-table. Through play the child will learn to express himself and to communicate with people, develop a social sense, gain experience and improved general development and a knowledge of everyday life.

REMEMBERING

This term means 'retaining past experiences'. It is a process which may vary in degree; for example, we may retain some previously learnt skill completely or in part.

Visualize the mind as a man living in a house which is surrounded by fields and has no road. At his front door he gets into his car and drives away, passing over the rough ground, leaving the impression of his car wheels. On his subsequent journeys he will follow his original tracks and will ultimately firmly define the path he takes by making the impressions deeper and deeper.

The marks first made represent a memory trace and the deepening of the first impression represents repetitive learning.

It is thought that in remembering, a memory trace is laid down on the mind, and being a sensory impression, by repetition the traces are made deeper and therefore more lasting. Once a memory trace is laid down it never completely disappears. The act of committing to memory consists of several processes :—

Registration.—This process is either active or passive. During a person's waking life, experiences are passively recorded on the mind as memory traces, some being deeper than others, depending upon the degree of emotional tension associated with them. Vivid experiences are more readily recorded than ordinary events of life and are more easily recalled.

Retentiveness.—Individuals show considerable differences in their power of retention. Some people are well known for their power of retaining knowledge (photographic memory).

We retain material that has been well understood better than poorly understood facts. Retention will depend to some extent on how effectively registration has been carried out ; interest in the task and concentration will improve registration. Practice, repetition, and recitation will also improve retention.

Recall.—The power to retain is not enough without the power to recall the memory traces laid down. Remembering cannot be said to have taken place unless past experiences can be recalled. A person who can recall past events as vividly as if they were actually taking place is said to have a good memory.

Recall is very sensitive to emotional stress. Some types of experiences which are acquired under severe emotional stress may be beyond the reach of voluntary recall and will require psychotherapy to bring them to the surface of the conscious mind.

The ability to recall can be improved by training.

Recognition.—What is recalled must be recognized as having occurred before ; in other words, the person must be familiar with the sensation.

Committing to Memory.—In a deliberate attempt to lay down memory traces for future recall it is better to have a general idea of the complete subject first and then fill in all the details afterwards. An actor learning his part in a play first of all reads the story through to gain an understanding of the plot, then he builds up an emotional impression around the character he has to portray in order to identify himself with it. From this beginning it will be easier to memorize the play.

Reading aloud lays down more new memory traces than does silent reading and assists in committing to memory.

Memory is impaired under certain conditions :—

1. Where there is excessive emotion.

2. In mental subnormality.

3. Damage to the brain cells where there is interference with the brain functions caused by trauma, bacteria, chemicals, senility, or general paralysis of the insane.

FORGETTING

This means 'failing to retain'. In fact, though the past experience cannot be recalled on demand as it were, the person will recognize it if subjected to the same stimulus or to associated stimuli.

To relearn a subject or skill is much easier than learning for the first time, which is a proof that memory traces last. Most people are required to learn a mass of information which is not going to be of use to them in their day-to-day living, and because these memory traces are not being used they are forgotten. To go back to the car-wheel impressions; if the car driver failed to use his car or used another track the original impressions would become overgrown and disappear from sight. This would take time and be a gradual process. It would become increasingly difficult to make out the impressions through the overgrowth. The impressions would remain, however, and could be exposed on removing the overgrowth. Far fewer journeys would be required to define the impressions firmly once again. So it is with relearning.

CHAPTER XXII

IMPRESSIONS

Sensation.—Sensation is apparent in the appreciation of environment. A person is usually conscious of what is in his environment. These contents produce stimuli which stimulate the sensory mechanism. Messages travel to the sensory part of the brain and there they create changes called ' sensory changes '.

There are several varieties of sensations which may be distinguished and can be divided into :—

1. The five special sensations of hearing, sight, smell, taste, and touch.

2. Organic sensations.

Though sensations are taking place all the time, a person is only paying attention to a few of them at a time.

Perception.—Paying attention to the detail of a sensation is called ' perception '.

Attention.—The producers of goods are constantly wanting the public to pay attention to their advertisements and to this end they display attractive posters advertising their products, frequently changing them to encourage people to increase their perceptions.

The factors concerned in attracting or increasing perception are :—

1. *Change.*—When walking, a person receives stimuli on the sole of the foot to which he pays no attention, but if the stimuli change, for instance, if he gets a stone in his shoe, he immediately becomes aware of the strength or power of the stimulus. The ticking of a clock in the room in which people reside is not noticed, but if the tick stops then the change is noticed.

2. *Change in Strength of the Stimulus.*—By this the strength of sensations may be compared. It varies with the degree of attention paid to it.

3. *Size of the Stimulus.*—Greater attention is demanded when two visual stimuli of a similar nature vary in size, or when there is something unusual about the stimuli, for example very tall or short persons. People of average height pass unnoticed.

4. *Repetition.*—The more frequently the stimulus is repeated the more likely is it to arrest attention. Mentally subnormals learn by repetition, which makes them pay more attention to the pronounced stimuli.

5. *Novelty.*—Anything that is new or unusual has a greater attraction than the everyday common thing. A stranger moving to a new town will quickly learn more about its history than the average local person who has spent the whole of his life there.

6. *Motives.*—Appeal to the motives, particularly the paternal, sex, and aggressive motives, will attract a person's attention.

7. *Emotion.*—Strong emotion makes a person pay more attention. A mother caring for her sick child pays no attention to outside noises, but if the sick child cries out she is immediately aware of it.

Any routine in the care of mentally subnormal persons should not be allowed to become monotonous, otherwise the repetition will bore the patient and he will lack interest and fail to learn.

Illusion.—This may be described as a wrong translation or perception of a sensory impression which takes place in the brain. The causes of illusions are :—

1. *Anxiety.*—A person in a house alone translates every noise as a burglar or someone breaking in.

2. *Fatigue.*—The senses being fatigued fail to take in the details of the impression and result in a wrong translation.

3. *Drugs.*—Morphine, phenobarbitone, alcohol, etc., dull the senses and depress their efficiency, resulting in false impressions.

In the normal and sane person illusions are quickly dispelled and corrected by further investigation and the use of reasoning power, but in the insane and the mentally subnormal very frequently impressions are misinterpreted, as when the patient describes the pattern of the wall-paper as faces which are watching him.

Hallucination.—This is a perception occurring in the absence of any sensation, in other words, a mental image or sensory impression without a sensory stimulus. The various types of hallucinations are : auditory (hearing), visual (sight), gustatory (taste), tactile (touch), and olfactory (smell).

Normal people suffer from mild forms of hallucinations when on the point of going to sleep. Sometimes a mental image of feeling the movement of a ship or hearing the sound of a train in motion, after having spent a considerable time travelling in one of these means of conveyance, persists for several hours.

Normal behaviour is to behave in an accepted normal way to stimulation. A person suffering from a mental disorder responds to his impression in a way that to him is normal, but is not considered normal by others in the community.

All behaviour is a result of mental impressions received from the environment, which appears completely different to different individuals.

A patient who behaves badly is, in his own idea, behaving quite rationally in response to his mental stimulus.

CHAPTER XXIII

PERSONALITY

THE personality of a man includes all his mental and physical characteristics. When these work together they enable him to react to his surroundings in a certain way.

Personality has been defined as "the most characteristic integration of an individual's physical structure, modes of behaviour, interests, attitudes, capacities, abilities and aptitudes". A personality trait is a particular quality such as honesty, aggressiveness, etc.

Though personality is a combination of every aspect of a human being, some aspects give more emphasis to the end-product than do others.

A person's physical appearance is important, as it does determine to a large degree how others react towards him, which in turn determines how he will react towards them.

If a person is said to have a good or pleasing personality it means he is liked by the person assessing him.

Temperament.—This is the habitual mental state characteristic of a person, which results from the influence upon the mind of several factors mostly related to bodily functions. These are : (1) Processes taking place inside the body, such as digestion and endocrine activity, which exert an influence upon the mental life and are thought to assist in shaping and determining individual temperaments ; (2) The degree of introversion or extroversion in attitudes of the mind.

The Introvert.—A person with this attitude of mind is the thoughtful type ; he is cool and deliberate, and never shows any emotional reactions ; he thinks before he acts. He finds his own amusements and interests, and is a poor mixer, preferring his own company to that of others.

The Extrovert.—This type of person displays quite the opposite characteristics. He is gay, cheerful, sociable, optimistic, and makes friends easily. He is more a practical minded person than a thinker. He is often impulsive, and will do things before considering the consequences of such action. He dislikes his own company and prefers to be with others. At times he may have mood-swings, sometimes being cheerful and at other times depressed and dejected.

Normally, temperament is inborn and fixed for each individual, but it may be modified by drugs, alcohol, and toxins.

Temperamental Types.—In the early days of psychology, psychologists classified the temperamental types as active ; sluggish ; tender ; and tough. Even earlier, humans were grouped as choleric (angry) ; sanguine (optimistic) ; phlegmatic (stolid) ; and melancholic (depressed).

In recent years temperamental variations have been associated with characteristic bodily structures. These are as follows :—

Pyknic.—The thick-set stocky person who in later life becomes fat. His temperament is cyclothymic, swinging from cheerfulness to depression, and he is much more likely to develop the manic-depressive psychosis if he suffers from mental illness. His mind and body are said to go in curves.

Athletic.—A big-boned, big-chested, and muscular person. His temperament is stable and not subjected to mood changes.

Asthenic.—The asthenic build is characterized by a pale, tall, thin, and narrow-chested person. His temperament is even in mood, but he is unsociable. Should he break down mentally he will tend towards a schizophrenic illness.

Understanding a person's temperamental make-up is of value in vocational guidance as well as in the rehabilitation of a mentally subnormal patient.

Disposition.—Disposition is said to be the result of the inborn variations in the strength of the motives, and a person may be said to have a timid disposition if the aggressive motive is weak, or an inquiring disposition if the curiosity motive is strong.

Character.—By character is meant the mental and moral equipment of a person which he acquires from his education and environment.   The inborn temperament and disposition enter into the formation of character.

Character is of slow growth.   It develops with all the other mental and physical characteristics.   To assess this attribute requires prolonged observation of a personal nature.

CHAPTER XXIV

THE UNCONSCIOUS MIND

THE central feature of the psychology of Freud, Jung, and Adler is the idea of the unconscious mind in the positive sense ; memories, experiences, etc., are forcibly held out of consciousness. The differences which exist between them are in what constitutes the unconscious mind and how material is held back from consciousness.

Freud described the mind as being in three parts :—

1. The Unconscious Mind (Subconscious).—The unconscious mind is that part of the mind where all thoughts and apparently forgotten impressions are put.

2. The Conscious Mind.—It is in the conscious mind that all one's thoughts are brought out into the open.

3. The Censor.—The censor lies between the conscious and subconscious mind and censors any of the thoughts wishing to pass into the conscious mind ; those which are approved of are allowed to pass to the higher level of the mind, the others are kept down in the unconscious mind.

It is claimed by some of the analytical schools that the unconscious mind is that part postulated by Freud as containing memory traces of which the individual is no longer aware.

During every moment of a man's waking life he is receiving impressions which he appears to ignore, and yet they pass through the conscious mind to the unconscious mind. Think of the ticking clock which suddenly stops. Up to the time it stops ticking, the tick is not being registered in the conscious mind, but the moment the ticking stops the conscious mind becomes aware of the change. The reason for the conscious mind's unawareness of the positive sensation is due to it passing straight through the conscious into the unconscious mind.

The Structure of the Mind.—

The Id.—Freud called the source of the infant's innate drives for food, sex, etc., the ' id '.

The id is egocentric, it does what it likes (pleasure principle) and avoids what it finds unpleasant (pain principle).

The Super Ego.—Restrictions are placed on the individual, and he has to accept the behaviour standards of people whose approval he values. The id is therefore restrained as reality impinges upon it. This part of the unconscious mind is called the ' super ego ' or ' conscience '.

The Ego.—The ego or self develops from the id. It is largely conscious and the term refers to that part of the personality of which the individual is usually aware.

The ego may be weak or strong. Ego weakness may result from a compulsion to expose oneself to stress together with an inability to cope with external factors.

If early relationships have been secure the personality is resistant to external stress and there is less compulsion to expose oneself to such stress—ego strength.

Conflict.—The meaning of conflict is ' a struggle of the mind ', which may be conscious or unconscious.

Whatever a person sets out to do he has first to make a decision, whether to do it or not to do it. Occasionally a struggle takes place between two opposing feelings or ideas, the desired one being conscious and the undesired one being subconscious. Until a decision is reached a conflict exists. Such a feeling may lead to disorders and disabilities in conduct.

When the ego is having difficulty in coping with problems, certain defence mechanisms (ego defences or mental mechanisms) come into operation.

Some of the mental mechanisms are : repression, regression, sublimation, projection, over-compensation, dissociation, rationalization.

Repression.—There are in us all instinctive wishes and strivings, many of which have to be restrained and controlled because of moral codes and social convention. Whenever the demands of society prevent the gratification of the instinctive wishes, a conflict is said to exist. In many individuals conscious resolution does not take place and because it is impossible to gratify the wish it is banished from the conscious mind and forms part of the unconscious mind and is then called a complex. Though this complex cannot be brought to the conscious mind voluntarily it does influence conscious thought and action.

The process of eliminating the complex from the conscious mind is termed ' repression '.

Regression.—Throughout life people undergo varying stages of development of behaviour, but at times of strain and illness some revert to one of the earlier stages of development. It is an unconscious retreat to a lower level of development.

Sublimation.—It is often necessary for a person to repress some of his sexual motives, but the driving force (libido) behind the motive which is being repressed is still active and causing unconscious conflict and frustration. A normal person will find for himself a suitable socially accepted and self-satisfying outlet for this energy, thus enriching his own personality and benefiting society. Athletics, dancing, social gatherings, and reading are some healthy activities which can be usefully applied to the act of sublimation.

Projection.—This is the mechanism by which experiences or ideas in a person's mind are unconsciously attributed to other people. A simple form of this mechanism affects most people at some time. Take yourself, for instance: if you become aware that you have a hole in the heel of your stocking, your mind not only dwells upon the hole, but you think that everyone else near you is noticing it, when in fact they have not seen it.

Over-compensation.—Normal compensation means that a person is putting enough effort forward to overcome a sense of inferiority or any physical defect which he may possess. Over-compensation is, however, an unconscious response which leads to the over-development of some other quality ; for example, an excessively shy person may over-compensate with boisterous behaviour.

Dissociation.—This mechanism may occur in varying degrees, from normal inconsistencies of conduct displayed in minor moral lapses to complete dissociation as found in mental illnesses. A person unconsciously refuses to recognize certain unpleasant items and may as a result forget large portions of his life. One frequently reads in the newspapers of the bridegroom-to-be who wanders away from his home a few hours before his wedding, forgetting that he is to be married and also who he is and where he lives (hysterical amnesia).

Rationalization.—Once a person has made a decision on the way he is going to behave in a given situation, he immediately makes excuses for this decision. The nurse who is studying for her examinations learns that there is a good film showing at the local cinema ; she knows that she should work if she wishes to pass the examinations, but she says to herself : "What I need is a change and a rest", and then goes off to the cinema. Rationalization is the mental process by which a plausible justification is made for something one wishes to believe or do, the real motive being subconscious.

Dreams.—After dreaming, one is usually able to describe what happened in detail. This is known as the ' manifest content '. To each dream there is a hidden meaning known as the ' latent content ', of which the manifest content is really the code.

During sleep the censor is not working as efficiently as it does during waking, and as a result all the thoughts and ideas resting in the unconscious mind try to get past the censor to reach the conscious mind.

Symbols.—Some of the thoughts and ideas do manage to reach consciousness in their original form, others pass disguised and are known as symbols or code. The actual form of their appearance is a substitution for the ideas repressed in the unconscious mind.

Displacement.—The apparent important content of the dream often turns out to be trivial when investigated, whilst those ideas and thoughts which are made to appear small and insignificant have important values.

Condensation.—The dream thoughts are a compact combination of many thoughts arising from the unconscious mind.

Dramatization.—The dream thoughts are arranged in such a way as to form a play which may be acted in a bizarre way leading to further concealment of the true meaning.

Dreams are usually quickly forgotten because once the censor becomes active and alert the dream contents are forced back into the unconscious mind.

CHAPTER XXV

EMOTIONS

VERY few motives are apparent in the young child ; most of them make their appearance at various stages of the infant's development. With the development of the principal motives there is also development of the accompanying states of feeling, such as fear, curiosity, anger, elation, etc., and to these states of feeling is given the name of emotion.

Although civilized man learns to control the actions to which he is prompted by his motives, he cannot avoid the emotions aroused by them. Take for instance the motive of pugnacity. Many people during the course of a lifetime have had this motivational urge stimulated, but owing to circumstances have acted with forbearance. In spite of the control exerted over the motive the emotion or feeling-tone of anger cannot be avoided ; it may persist for several hours, and influence a man's behaviour towards his work, other people, and inanimate objects.

Accompanying mental development is a blending of primary emotions which gives rise to complex emotional states ; for example, the blending together of the primary emotions of wonder and subjection produces the emotion of admiration.

With a higher degree of mental development further complicated blending of emotions takes place, producing more complex emotional states. From the grouping of these complex feeling-tones sentiments are formed.

EMOTIONAL DEVELOPMENT

From the very beginning of postnatal life the child experiences internal sensations of pain, pressure, hunger, heat, cold, and muscle movement. The first intense sensations are connected with the processes of feeding and eliminating waste products.

The most marked emotions during infancy are affection and anger. Affection towards the mother is first shown by the infant's little patting, stroking, and handling movements of her body.

While the baby is sucking at his mother's breast he is satisfying a very intense craving and gaining a pleasant emotion from the experience. A disturbance of the activity will usually produce a tempestuous reaction demonstrated by screaming, kicking, and punching, which are forms of retaliation and represent the first characteristic expression of anger.

The frustration of a desire and deprivation of a satisfaction produce an intense expression and a feeling of anger and hate which is liable to occur throughout childhood. Anger in infancy quickly changes to affection when the desire is satisfied. The infant feels that the person who satisfies him is good and lovable.

Babies suck their thumbs as a substitute for the breast and endeavour to reproduce the pleasurable sensations of breast-feeding. Sucking, when proceeding harmoniously, provides the infant with satisfaction, contentment, security, and happiness. It is important that the baby has sufficient food and is not left with a feeling of hunger after a feed.

Emotional excitement tends to occur at any time when bodily changes or stimulation take place. Under ordinary conditions emotion is simply an organic preparedness for activity. The organic changes which take place prepare the body for harmonious action.

During early life the child has relatively little control over his emotional stresses, and the intensity of his emotional outbursts is extreme and can fluctuate from one emotion to another. Most of these storms are centred around his parents.

After the age of 5 years, most children develop a degree of control over their emotions, and this control strengthens with the progress of life and as a result of adequate training. The child learns to accept frustrations and disappointments more willingly than he did before.

Having developed a greater degree of security in life through his experiences, he develops a decreasing dependency on his parents and because of this his conflict of feeling towards them is less intense and more rational.

The child does, however, develop an attitude of being less willing to confide in his parents and does indeed become more hostile and rebellious towards them, but without it coming to such a degree as to mar all his relationships with his father and mother.

As the child grows older he will form close friendships with people outside his own family circle, and these friendships assist in the promotion of satisfactory emotional development. Because of jealousy and hostility the bonds of friendship will periodically be broken and be as easily mended again. Moods will fluctuate in frequency and degree.

Children of around 11 years of age find a great source of confidence and security in their group associations (clubs and associations) and in return they pledge their loyalty to their group.

It is at the age of 11 that imitative behaviour and loyalty can, if not directed into the correct channels, become uncontrollable delinquent behaviour with its catastrophic destruction of a useful life, and parental distress.

The period of adolescence, though interesting, is not easy for a young person. There is an increase in emotional strain, self-consciousness, and a loss of self-assurance, with an awakening of sexual desire. These produce swinging moods of elation and despair, which may be intense.

The return of day-dreaming is characteristic of this age-period. Reality is completely blotted out by the dreams of being rich, popular, and capable of performing great feats of heroism. The child is trying to find a substitute for the reality.

The adolescent is most critical of his parents and feels defiant towards their authority. This is a natural process of development and represents the last stage of the weaning process from his dependency on his parents. Once he has passed through this stage of emotional eruption he settles down to enjoy more stable relationships with his parents. Once more he will seek their advice and listen to them with respect. He withdraws from the gangs he has previously been loyal to, and in their place he forms deep attachments, at first with people of the same sex and later with someone of the opposite sex. Though these love affairs are immature they do form trial grounds for adult love, and later, marriage and parenthood.

EMOTIONAL MATURITY

On reaching adulthood a man has reached the peak of his physical powers, and if his psychological development has passed normally through all the normal stages, he will have reached a stage of maturity which will assist him to adjust his life to the demands of social intercourse, personal relationships, work, marriage, and parenthood. Though the person has reached emotional maturity he will still be subjected to great emotional stress, often of a greater degree than in his younger immature life, but to the normal stable person none of these stresses is likely to prove intolerable.

Courtship between two members of the opposite sex, though providing a greater satisfaction than any other kind of human relationship, makes greater demands, especially in the early stages of courtship when there are heightened sensibilities created by the emotion of love.

Marriage for most people is the most happy and satisfying period, both emotionally and physically, of their whole lives. The process of adjusting two lives to harmonize with each other, though often delicate and complicated, is made easy and pleasurable by the happiness of mutual love.

Starting a family demands more re-adjustment and an acceptance of heavier responsibilities. Even in the most mature relationship, parenthood inevitably calls for great emotional adjustment.

At first glance it seems that the father does not enter into the parent–child relationship and this oneness between mother and baby can create tensions where adjustments are not adequate.

EMOTION AS A FACTOR IN DISEASE

Psychosomatic medicine has focused attention upon emotion as a causative factor in many diseases, including the well-recognized gastro-intestinal disorders.

Prolonged emotional upsets do appear to be related to the onset of organic disease. It has been found that anxiety prolongs digestion and that lesser emotions can also affect it ; as an example, the anticipation of a favourite food will stimulate the secretion of gastric juices, whereas food which looks unpleasant and is served in smelly, dirty surroundings will retard digestion.

The basal metabolism is raised by emotional stress, and differences have been found between normal and emotionally disordered individuals.

Emotional reaction results in an outpouring of adrenaline which hastens the clotting of blood, stimulates an increased output of red blood-cells, and through its action upon the spleen, causes it to contract and increase the volume of blood.

Anxiety is usually accompanied by an increased cardiac output which may be associated with an increased pulse-rate.

During sleep which is being disturbed by dreams the blood-pressure will rise, and if the rise affects a person already subjected to hypertension, the pressure will rise higher and will last longer.

Afflictions of the skin, which are common amongst emotionally disturbed individuals, take many forms and appear to deteriorate with each emotional stress.

In health, emotions are rarely experienced without there being a situation present which has invoked them. When a person experiences fear it is because of something in his environment which has suddenly destroyed his feeling of security.

The emotions have a very strong survival value ; at the same time as the emotional experience takes place, an impulse to react is generated.

The most vital driving force behind human behaviour is emotion, and when the capacity for emotional experience is lost, activity and the capacity to react with feeling are lost also.

263

BIBLIOGRAPHY

ABEL-SMITH, B. (1960), *A History of the Nursing Profession.* London: Heinemann.
— — (1965), *The Hospitals 1800–1948: A Study in Social Administration in England and Wales.* London: Heinemann.
BALINT, M. (1961), *Psychotherapeutic Techniques in Medicine.* London: Tavistock.
BANTON, M. (1965), *Roles.* London: Tavistock.
BARTON, R. (1966), *Institutional Neurosis,* 2nd ed. Bristol: Wright.
BERGER, J. (1967), *Fortunate Man.* Harmondsworth: Penguin.
BIESTEK, F. P. (1965), *Casework Relationship.* London: Allen & Unwin.
Lord BRAIN (1965), *Speech Disorders: Aphasia, Apraxia and Agnosia,* 2nd ed. London: Butterworths.
BURR, J. (1968), *Swire's Handbook of Practical Nursing,* 6th ed. London: Baillière, Tindall & Cassell.
BUSS, A. H. (1961), *Psychology of Aggression.* New York: Wiley.
CANDLAND, D. K. (1968), *Psychology: The Experimental Approach.* New York: McGraw-Hill.
CAPLAN, G. (1961), *Community Approach to Mental Health.* London: Tavistock.
— — (1961), *Prevention of Mental Disorders in Children.* London: Tavistock.
— — (1965), *Principles of Preventive Psychiatry.* London: Tavistock.
CASH, J. E. (1965), *A Textbook of Medical Conditions for Physiotherapists,* 3rd ed. London: Faber.
CATTERALL, R. D. (1965), *A Short Textbook of Venereology.* London: E.U.P.
Cerebellum, Posture and Cerebral Palsy (1963). National Spastics Society Medical Education and Information Unit.
CUMMING, J., and CUMMING, E. (1962), *Ego and Milieu.* London: Tavistock.
EASTHAM, R. D., and JANCAR, J. (1968), *Clinical Pathology in Mental Retardation.* Bristol: Wright.
ELLIS, N. R. (1963), *Handbook of Mental Deficiency.* New York: McGraw-Hill.
FEDERMAN, D. D. (1967), *Abnormal Sexual Development: A Genetic and Endocrine Approach to Differential Diagnosis.* Philadelphia: Saunders.
FERARD, M. L. (1962), *The Caseworker's Use of Relationships.* London: Tavistock. Philadelphia: Lippincott.
FLETCHER, H. (1953), *Speech and Hearing in Communication.* New York: Van Nostrand.

FOULDS, G. A. (1965), *Personality and Personal Illness.* London: Tavistock.
FREEMAN, T., and others (1965), *Studies on Psychosis.* London: Tavistock.
FRIEDMAN, L. J. (1962), *Virgin Wives.* London: Tavistock.
GOLDBERG, E. M. (1958), *Family Influences and Psychosomatic Illness.* London: Tavistock.
GOODE, W. J. (1964), *The Family.* New York: Prentice-Hall.
Guidance to Parents of Deaf Children (1966). London: Pitman Medical.
GUNTRIP, H. (1964), *Healing the Sick Mind.* London: Allen & Unwin.
HEATON-WARD, W. A. (1967), *Mental Subnormality,* 3rd ed. Bristol: Wright.
HENDERSON, Sir D., and BATCHELOR, I. R. C. (ed.) (1962), *Henderson and Gillespie's Text-book of Psychiatry,* 9th ed. London: O.U.P.
HOCHBERG, J. (1964), *Perception.* New York: Prentice-Hall.
HORDER, M. (1966), *The Little Genius.* London: Duckworth.
HUNTER, R., and MACALPINE, I. (1963), *Three Hundred Years of Psychiatry, 1385–1860: A History Presented in Selected English Texts.* London: O.U.P.
JOLLY, H. (1968), *Diseases of Children,* 2nd ed. Oxford: Blackwell.
KENYON, F. C. (1968), *Psychiatric Emergencies and the Law.* Bristol: Wright.
LAING, R. D. (1964), *Reason and Violence.* London: Tavistock.
LORING, J. (1966), *Teaching the Cerebral Palsied Child.* London: National Spastics Society in association with Heinemann.
LURIA, A. R., and YODOVICH, F. I. (1959), *Speech and the Development of Mental Processes in the Child.* London: Staples Press.
McDOWAL, E. B. (1964), *Teaching the Severely Subnormal.* London: Arnold.
McGHEE, A. (1966), *Psychology applied to Nursing,* 4th ed. London: Macmillan.
McKEOWN, T., and LOWE, C. R. (1966), *An Introduction to Social Medicine.* Oxford: Blackwell Scientific.
MACNAB, F. A. (1965), *Estrangement and Relationship.* London: Tavistock.
MASTERS, W. H., and JOHNSON, V. E. (1966), *Human Sexual Response.* Boston: Little, Brown.
MEDNICK, S. A. (1964), *Learning.* New York: Prentice-Hall.
Motor Deficit (1965). National Spastics Society Medical Education and Information Unit.
O'CONNOR, N., and TIZARD, J. (1956), *Social Problems of Mental Deficiency.* Oxford: Pergamon.
PALMER, J. O., and GOLDSTEIN, M. J. (ed.) (1966), *Perspectives in Psychopathology: Readings in Abnormal Psychology.* London: O.U.P.
PENROSE, L. S. (1934), *The Influence of Heredity.* London: Lewis.
— — (1964), *The Biology of Mental Defect,* 3rd ed. London: Sidgwick & Jackson.
PHILP, A. F. (1963), *Family Failure.* London: Faber.
REES, W. L. L. (1967), *A Short Textbook of Psychiatry.* London: E.U.P.
ROBERTS, J. A. F. (1967), *An Introduction to Medical Genetics,* 4th ed. London: O.U.P.

RUDD, T. N. (1966), *The Elderly Sick*, 5th ed. London: Faber.
— — (1967), *Human Relations in Old Age*. London: Faber.
SHIRLEY, H. F. (1963), *Paediatric Psychiatry*. Cambridge, Mass: Harvard U.P.
SIMEONS, A. T. W. (1966), *Man's Presumptuous Brain*. London: Longmans.
SINGTON, D. (1964), *Psychosocial Aspects of Drug-taking*. Oxford: Pergamon.
SLAUGHTER, S. S. (1960), *The Mentally Retarded Child and His Parent*. New York: Harper & Row.
SODDY, K. (1967), *Men in Middle Life*. London: Tavistock. Philadelphia: Lippincott.
— — and AHRENFELDT, R. H. (ed.) (1967), *Mental Health and Contemporary Thought*. London: Tavistock. Philadelphia: Lippincott.
— — — — (1964), *Mental Health in the Service of the Community*. London: Tavistock. Philadelphia: Lippincott.
— — — — (1965), *Mental Health in a Changing World*. London: Tavistock.
STOTT, D. H. (1966), *Studies of Troublesome Children*. London: Tavistock.
SUSSER, M. W., and WATSON, W. (1962), *Sociology in Medicine*. London: O.U.P.
Lord TAYLOR and CHAVE, S. (1964), *Mental Health and Environment*. London: Longmans.
THORNE, G. D. (1965), *Understanding the Mentally Retarded*. New York: McGraw-Hill.
TIZARD, J. (1964), *Community Services for the Mentally Handicapped*. London: O.U.P.
TOD, R. J. N. (1968), *Children in Care*, vol. 1. London: Longmans.
TREDGOLD, R. F., and SODDY, K. (1963), *Textbook of Mental Deficiency*, 10th ed. London: Baillière, Tindall & Cassell.
TREVELYAN, G. M. (1946), *English Social History*, 3rd ed. London: Longmans.
WALE, J. O. (ed.) (1968), *Tidy's Massage and Remedial Exercises*, 11th ed. Bristol: Wright.
WATTS, C. A. H. (1966), *Depressive Disorders in the Community*. Bristol: Wright.
WERKMEN, S. L. (1966), *The Role of Psychiatry in Medical Education*. Cambridge, Mass.: Harvard U.P.
WHITLOCK, F. A. (1963), *Criminal Responsibility and Mental Illness*. London: Butterworths.
WRIGHT, F. R. (1966), *Parallels of Power*. Bristol: Wright.
YOUNGHUSBAND, E. L. (1965), *Social Work and Families*, vol. 1. London: National Institute for Social Work Training.

266

APPENDIX

NOTES ON THE ENGLISH AND SCOTTISH MENTAL HEALTH ACTS

BY RICHARD SHORT, L.R.C.P. & S., L.R.F.P.S., D.P.H.

Medical Officer for Mental Health Services to the City of Edinburgh

ADMINISTRATIVELY, the Old Acts were designed for very different conditions from the present, when the vast majority of the patients concerned are wholly or partly under the care of the National Health Service. The terminology was also out of date, and some of the underlying concepts were no longer in accord with modern ideas and advances in medicine.

In 1954 a Royal Commission was appointed to consider, as regards England and Wales, the law relating to mental illness and mental deficiency. The Commission made its report in 1957 and the Scottish Health Services Council subsequently considered and reported on the application to Scotland of the major recommendations.

The Mental Health Act, 1959, for England and Wales, and the Mental Health (Scotland) Act, 1960, which followed these reports sought to ensure that, wherever possible, the mentally disordered patient can have the same ready access, without formality, to care and treatment as the patient suffering from some physical disorder. Special safeguards are provided to protect patients whose care and treatment must be under conditions of compulsory detention. It also extends to mentally disordered persons, according to the conditions under which they are treated or cared for, the special measures of protection which they require because they are not always able to protect themselves and their own interests.

The Scottish Act differs materially from the English Act in the following points :—

Terminology.—Mental Disorder is used in both Acts to cover all forms of mental ill-health, including mental deficiency.

The English Act also gives four main categories of mentally disordered patients :—

1. Mental illness.
2. Severe subnormality—means a state of arrested or incomplete development of mind which includes subnormality of intelligence and is of such a nature or degree that the patient is incapable of living an independent life or of guarding himself against serious exploitation, or will be so incapable when of an age to do so.

3. Subnormality—means a state of arrested or incomplete development of mind (not amounting to severe subnormality) which includes subnormality of intelligence and is of a nature or degree which requires or is susceptible to medical treatment or other special care or training of the patient.

4. Psychopathic disorder—means a persistent disorder or disability of mind which results in abnormally aggressive or serious irresponsible conduct on the part of the patient, and requires or is susceptible to medical treatment or care or training under medical supervision.

Scottish Act—only two categories given :—

1. Mental illness.

2. Mental deficiency : This category is not defined in the Scottish Act. The definition is, however, generally regarded as social in nature, although psychometrically the upper level for compulsory admission or guardianship is at about the 70 per cent level on the intelligence quotient scale (*see also p. 268,* ' Exceptions ').

Procedure for Admission to Hospital.—There is nothing to prevent a patient from being admitted to any hospital or nursing home and receiving treatment there without any of the formal procedures set out in the Act, i.e., can be admitted as patients normally admitted to hospital for treatment of physical conditions.

English Act.—Methods of compulsory admission :—

1. Admission for observation (Section 25).

2. Emergency admission for observation (Section 29).

3. Admission for treatment (Section 26).

4. Reception into guardianship (Section 33).

5. Admission on court order (Section 60).

6. Admission by Home Office transfer.

7. Admission on removal from Scotland or N. Ireland.

Scottish Act.—No compulsory admission for observation. The Dunlop Committee in considering this point stated as follows :—

" We have considered the Royal Commission's suggestions that it would be helpful to have compulsory powers available by which mentally ill patients and high-grade mental defectives could be admitted to hospital for up to 28 days' observation and preliminary treatment. We have reached the conclusion that this suggestion should not be adopted in Scotland in respect of the mentally ill : our reasons are as follows :—

" (a) We consider that our proposals for facilitating voluntary admission reduce in substantial measure the case for introduction of the 28-days' period.

"(b) The suggested procedure could benefit only relatively few patients, whereas, if misused, it could work to the detriment of many.

"(c) We could not contemplate the introduction of such a procedure without the participation in it of the sheriff, and a judicial order for a restricted period would not appear to have much point."

In the *Scottish Act,* therefore, compulsory admission is limited to :—

1. Admission for treatment (Section 24).
2. Emergency admission for treatment (Section 31).
3. Reception into guardianship (Sections 24, 33).
4. Admission on court order.
5. Admission by Secretary of State transfer.
6. Admission on removal from England and Wales to Scotland.

PROCEDURE

In dealing with procedure, reference is made to compulsory admissions to hospital or guardianship and not to court admissions, etc.

England and Wales.—Application is made for a patient's compulsory hospital admission or guardianship of Local Health Authority by a relative or a Mental Welfare Officer of the Local Health Authority with the support of two medical recommendations, but without reference to a judicial authority.

Scotland.—As for England, but the application must be approved by the Sheriff.

Reasons given by the Royal Commission against the need for a judicial authority were that there was not much safeguard for a patient in putting facts before a Magistrate ; that it was a relic of the " police " and poor law powers and that it linked mental treatment with the punishment of crime. Safeguard is now afforded by local " Review Tribunals ". On the other hand, the Scottish Commission contended that it seemed wrong, where it was proposed to deprive a person of his liberty, that no person or body other than the doctors should participate in dealing with the application.

Exceptions.—Both Acts contain provisos relating to age and mental disorder.

The Scottish Act states that no person over the age of 21 years shall be compulsorily admitted except where :—

1. The mental deficiency is such that he is incapable of living an independent life or of guarding himself against serious exploitation ; or
2. Mental illness is other than a persistent disorder which is manifested only by abnormally aggressive or seriously irresponsible conduct.

A patient who has been in these classes admitted before the age of 21 years will not be liable to detention or guardianship after the age of 25 years unless likely to act dangerously.

The English Act contains similar provisions but allows psychopaths to be liable to compulsory admission to hospital for medical observation at any age, provided that they are not compulsorily detained for longer than 28 days.

In the case of formal procedure one of the medical recommendations must be made by a doctor approved by a Regional Hospital Board as having special experience in the diagnosis or treatment of mental disorder. In England the doctor must be approved by the Local Health Authority.

In Scotland the Local Health Authority officer is called the Mental Health Officer and in England the Mental Welfare Officer. In making an application a Mental Health Officer must see the case within 14 days before making the application.

EMERGENCY PROCEDURE

England and Wales and Scotland.—An emergency recommendation may be made by a medical practitioner who has personally examined the patient on the day on which he signed the recommendation. An emergency recommendation shall not be made unless, where practicable, the consent of a relative or a Mental Health Officer (England : Mental Welfare Officer) has been obtained ; and the recommendation shall be accompanied by a statement that such consent has been obtained, or by a statement giving reasons for failure to obtain the consent.

The only difference between the two Acts is that of time. In the English Act another doctor must be called within 72 hours if the patient's detention is to go on longer than that. In Scotland the recommendation authorizes the removal of the patient *within* 72 hours from the date on which it was made and for his detention therein for a period not exceeding 7 days.

DURATION OF DETENTION

The authority to detain in hospital for treatment or to keep under guardianship will lapse at the end of a year, but it may be renewed for a year, and on subsequent expiry for periods of 2 years if the Responsible Medical Officer reports that this is necessary in the interests of the patient's health or safety.

Supervision and Appeals.—In Scotland appeals can be made by the patient or relatives to the Sheriff, and the Mental Welfare Commission replaces the Board of Control in its supervisory capacity. These tribunals are constituted for every Hospital Region and consist of legal, medical, and lay members having experience in administration or knowledge of social services, and are appointed by the Lord Chancellor. In England and Wales the Review Tribunal is the authority for appeals.

FUNCTIONS OF LOCAL HEALTH AUTHORITIES

1. The Provision, Equipment, etc., of Residential Accommodation.—

One of the general principles which the Royal Commission laid down for the future was that there should be an increasing emphasis on care in the community, rather than institutional care, for all those suffering from mental illness or mental deficiency who were not in need of the special facilities which the hospital service offered for in-patients. The Scottish Committee supported this principle and emphasized the need to allow mentally disordered patients to enter into the life of the community as far as their disability would allow.

Local Authority Residential Accommodation could thus be used to reduce the need for hospital admission for those not in the community and enable hospital in-patients to return to the community after as short a period of hospital treatment as possible.

The accommodation has also to be adapted to meet the needs of the two groups of mental disorder, as it is currently felt that it is unwise to mix the mental defectives and the mentally ill patients.

Mental Defectives—Accommodation.—The needs for residential accommodation for the mental defectives are :—

    a. Short-term Homes.

    b. Longer-term Hostels for School-age Children.

    c. Residential Accommodation for Adults.

    a. Short-term Homes : Short-stay homes for both adults and children have as their object the relief for those looking after them during periods of domestic stress or for holidays. In some cases arrangements may be made for temporary admission to a mental deficiency hospital, or where the demand is limited by local authorities combining to establish a joint provision. The solution in some areas may be through a voluntary association.

    b. Longer-term Hostels for School-age Children : The children for whom such centres would cater are those whose defect is too severe to make them suitable for an education authority residential school or occupation centre, who cannot receive occupational training at home, and yet do not necessarily require treatment in hospital. This type of home is more suited to a country area where those children are not within reach of a day centre.

Hospitals, however, should remain responsible for those children who appear likely to require constant and close supervision throughout life and who will never be able to take any significant part in the life of the community.

    c. Residential Accommodation for Adults : Mental defectives who can obtain outside employment may need special accommodation in a hostel either because they are homeless and cannot in the ordinary way find suitable lodgings, or particularly in the case of school leavers, young adults and mental defectives leaving hospital because they need for a time more supervision than they can receive at home or in lodgings. Hostels should be near the centre of employment.

Such a hostel may be at or near a sheltered workshop or training centre for those who cannot obtain open employment immediately and who require a period of training.

There may also be a need of accommodation for mental defectives who are incapable of ordinary employment, unsuitable for boarding-out with individual guardians and without homes in the community. But where such persons require close and constant supervision and *are incapable of taking any significant part in the life of the community*—they should remain in hospital. There may be mental defectives living in the community who fall into the above category on the death of parents or relatives. It is suggested by the Advisory Committee that these cases should be given special consideration by the Local Authority for long-term accommodation in its hostels as an alternative to admission to hospital.   Such hostels are said to be desirable particularly for aged mental defectives.

Mentally Ill—Accommodation.—It is not anticipated that the demand for the mentally ill will be great and they will probably have to meet the need of patients who have been in hospital for some considerable time and who will have to re-adjust themselves slowly to normal life in the community.

Lodgings : It is suggested by the Advisory Committee that suitable lodgings for patients leaving mental hospitals should be found and that the Local Authority could assist in this field.

Homes for Old People : There is a need for homes for certain aged mentally disturbed patients.   It is suggested that these homes should be small and they can be provided either under the National Assistance Act, through the welfare authority, or under the National Health Service and Mental Health Acts.

Short-term Residential Accommodation : It is considered that there is a need for short-term accommodation for mentally ill patients in periods of domestic stress or to give those looking after them a holiday.   This could be provided either through the hospital service, in suitable lodgings, or a Local Authority hostel.

Accommodation for Children : The effect of the new Act is that the Local Authority, as children's authority, may admit to children's homes and other accommodation provided by them under the Children Act, mentally disordered children who have not been received into care under that Act, but who are receiving care under the National Health Service Act.   This enables the Local Authority to set aside certain homes or separate parts of homes for mentally disordered children.

2.   Appointment of Mental Welfare Officers (England and Wales), or Mental Health Officers (Scotland).—

In the terms of the new Acts, Local Health Authorities are required to appoint Mental Welfare or Health Officers whose statutory duties may be compared with those of the " authorized officer " under the old legislation, and they set in motion the procedure for compulsory admission to hospital or reception into guardianship where this is necessary, and the patient's relatives are unable or unwilling to take action.

In addition to his statutory duties, the Mental Welfare or Health Officer may be employed in the care and after-care of patients living in the community or discharged from hospital, and practical work is likely to include helping patients with their financial and employment problems by negotiating with the various bodies and employers.   Their work is likely to be complementary to the health visitors' care of patients in the community.

3.   Guardianship.—

Mental Defectives.—Local Health Authorities already have power, under the National Health Service Act, to provide informal supervision of mental defectives, but the new Act for the first time specifically refers to " the supervision " by Local Health Authorities—" of persons suffering from mental deficiency who are neither liable to detention in a hospital nor subject to guardianship ". At the same time, the Act makes it plain that before a patient can be received into formal guardianship it must be " necessary in the interests of the health and safety of the patients or for the protection of other persons that the patient should be so received ". This in effect means that the doctors and the Sheriff (in Scotland) who approve the application must be satisfied that there is no other satisfactory way of dealing with the patient in the community. It will therefore not be possible to place a patient under formal guardianship if informal supervision is sufficient to provide him with the care and treatment that he needs.

Mentally Ill.—Guardianship under the new Act also applies to mentally ill patients as well as to mental defectives or subnormals and the provisions for admission to formal guardianship under the supervision of the Local Health Authority are similar. At present it is very rare for mentally ill patients to be boarded out in private dwellings direct : most of those at present boarded out are patients who have been in a mental hospital, have subsequently been discharged on probation, but who were not considered fit for full discharge after a year on probation, although they could remain in the community.

4. Ancillary or Supplementary Services.—

This can cover a very wide variety of services, ranging from social work for the mentally disordered to the provision of medical and dental services for the mentally disordered children who are not able to attend school. Day centres for the elderly patients and social clubs for the elderly, mentally ill, patients, and mental defectives come within this heading.

5. Ascertainment of Mental Deficiency.—

The term ascertainment is used in the sense of " assessing the need " and not in the educational sense of assessing the intelligence quotient and educability. The Local Health Authority's duty includes children of pre-school age, but excludes children of school age because the Education Authority has a duty to ascertain children of school age who need special educational treatment or whose disability of mind is such that they are unsuitable for education or training in a special school.

Hitherto the Local Health Authority's duty of ascertainment was confined to defectives in respect of whom compulsory action was necessary. Now the responsibility is wider, and it is concerned rather to discover all those persons in their area who by reason of mental deficiency or subnormality may be in need of and capable of benefiting from the services which they have to offer.

Pre-school Child.—The existing Child Welfare and Health Visiting Services usually bring to the notice of a Health Department any child suffering from mental deficiency. The aim must be to ensure that the services are such that no child in need of treatment, training, or other special help because of mental disability can escape their notice.

It is advised that general practitioners should be asked to consult the Local Health Authority before the child reaches the age of 3 years about any case in which there may be mental handicap. It is also important for

Health Visitors to see all children in their districts between the ages of 2 and 3 years. Where, as a result of a visit, there is reason to suspect mental handicap, it is suggested that the Medical Officer of Health should write to the child's general practitioner to ask if he would wish himself to arrange for the necessary investigation or whether the Local Authority should carry out the investigation.

Specialist diagnostic services should be provided and these could be in Local Health Authority premises staffed in part from the hospital service.

Under the Education Act, parents may ask the Education Authority to examine a child between the ages of 2 and 5 years, with a view to the ascertainment of mental or physical handicap. If the Education Authority then decide that the child, even at that age, is clearly not going to be suitable for education within the school system, they are able to report the child formally to the Local Health Authority without waiting until he reaches the age of 5 years.

School-age Child.—If the Education Authority decide that a child is "ineducable" (England and Wales), or "untrainable" (Scotland), they have a duty to report the child to the Local Health Authority. In addition, it is recommended that the Local Health Authority should be informed of any child who, while capable of receiving education, might benefit from informal supervision.

The Education Authority has hitherto had a duty to inform the Local Health Authority of any child who is suffering from a disability of mind of such a nature or to such an extent that he may require to be dealt with under the Mental Deficiency Acts after leaving school. This is now replaced by the much wider duty to report to the Local Health Authority any child who is suffering from mental deficiency to such an extent that he may, on leaving school, benefit from the services which the Local Health Authority has power to provide.

Assessment of Needs of Adults.—This can be done through co-operation with the various statutory and voluntary bodies.

6. Informal Supervision.—

It should be the aim of the Local Health Authority under the new Act to provide advice and visits to all mental defectives in the community and to all those looking after them who need it and desire it, whether under guardianship or not. Reference has already been made to the fact that guardianship can only be considered when informal visitation is not sufficient to meet the interests of the patient or for the protection of other persons.

7. Training and Occupation for Children under 16 Years and for Persons over 16 Years.—

The Acts make no change in the scope of the present duties of Local Health Authorities and Education Authorities with regard to the training and occupation of mentally handicapped children and adult mental defectives.

A duty is placed on the Local Health Authority to provide transport where it thinks it necessary to enable persons to receive occupation and

19

training. This applies whether the occupation and training is provided directly by the Local Health Authority or by arrangements with voluntary organizations or other departments of the Local Authority. This section includes the refund of travelling expenses in appropriate cases.

Enforcement of Attendance at Training and Occupation Centres.—The Local Health Authority has a new power to require attendance at an occupation centre of children under 16 years who have been reported as ineducable and untrainable at a special school.

8. Services under the National Assistance Act.—

Local Authorities may accommodate a person with any degree of mental disorder in a welfare home provided under the National Assistance Act. Homes for the aged mentally disturbed patients may therefore be provided under the National Health Service Act or the National Assistance Act.

Under the new Act, mental disability is extended to cover persons suffering from mental disorder of any description. This overcomes the limitations imposed by the wording of the National Assistance Act which relates to services for " those whose disability is such as to cause a substantial and permanent handicap ".

9. Child Care Services.—

Local Authorities have the discretion to provide services for mentally disordered children within the framework of either their child care services or other health services, whichever seems appropriate to the circumstances of any individual case.

Visiting of Patients in Hospital.—The Act requires a Local Authority, which is acting as parent, guardian, or nearest relative to a mentally disordered patient under certain statutory provisions, to maintain contact with the patient if he enters a hospital or nursing home in Scotland for any form of treatment, by arranging visits or taking such other steps as might be expected of a parent.

INDEX